5 minute HAIR

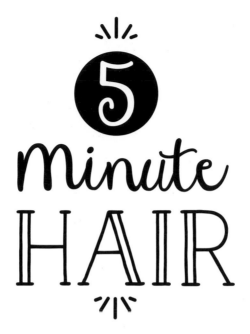

'To my children. May you always have the confidence to chase your dreams.'

An Hachette UK Company
www.hachette.co.uk

First published in Great Britain in 2016 by Mitchell Beazley, an imprint of Octopus Publishing Group Ltd, Carmelite House, 50 Victoria Embankment, London, EC4Y 0DZ
www.octopusbooks.co.uk

A CIP catalogue record for this book is available from the British Library.

ISBN 978-1-7847-2243-2

This book was conceived, designed and produced by The Bright Press, an imprint of The Quarto Group. The Old Brewery, 6 Blundell Street, London N7 9BH, United Kingdom.
(0)20 7700 6700 www.QuartoKnows.com

Publisher: Mark Searle
Editorial Director: Isheeta Mustafi
Commissioning Editor: Alison Morris
Editor: Angela Koo
Junior Editor: Abbie Sharman
Art Director: Michelle Rowlandson
Design concept: Michelle Rowlandson
Book layout: Agata Rybicka and Richard Peters
Cover design: Michelle Rowlandson
Photographer: Sara Bishop

10 9 8 7 6 5 4 3

Printed in China by Toppan Leefung

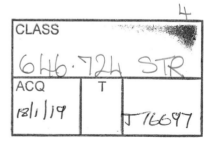

Cover Credits:
Front (top to bottom, left to right): Getty Images; Photography by Sara Bishop, styling by Jenny Strebe, model Alexia Poisot; Getty Images.
Bottom (top to bottom): Photography by Sara Bishop, styling by Jenny Strebe, models Mallory Jarvis, Jacque Stuard, Jasmine Jacobson, Shelby Barnes.

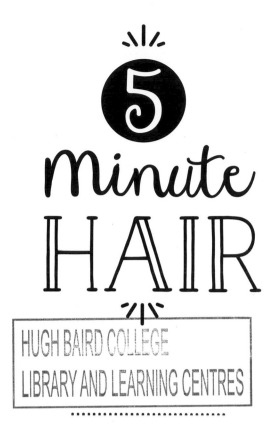

5 minute HAIR

50 super-quick hairstyles to wear and go

JENNY STREBE

MITCHELL
BEAZLEY

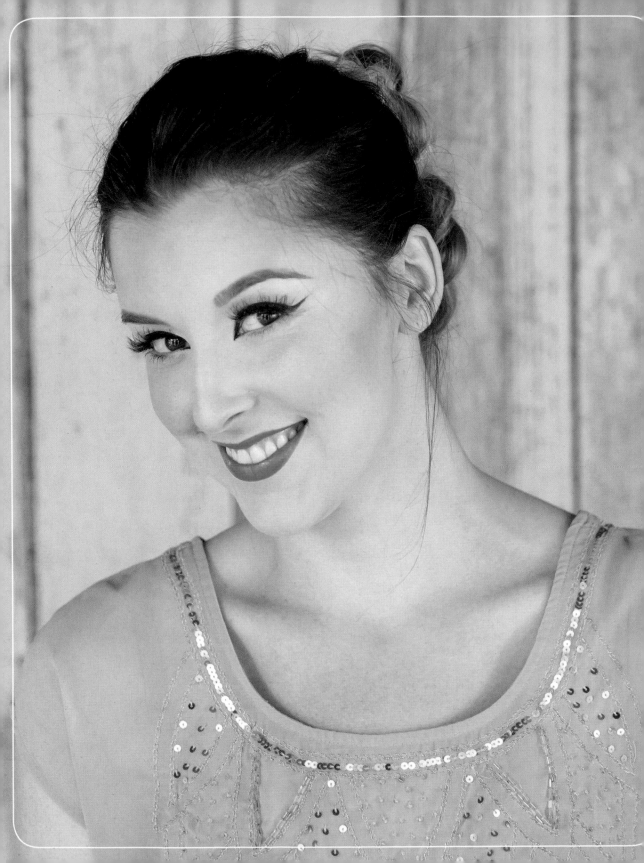

CONTENTS

Double-plaited bun, pages 62–63

INTRODUCTION

 Through the process of creating books and travelling to different salons for meet-and-greets, book signings and classes, I have learnt many valuable hair tricks. One of these tricks is the art of creating a great hairstyle in very little time. So, to share the benefits of my experience with you, I have interpreted my own hairstyles to come up with a collection of looks that can be created in under five minutes!

I created this book with a typical girl on the go in mind. Sometimes life gets crazy and you need a look that will fit your needs throughout the day. The one thing you want but just don't have is time. Well, that and a pair of comfortable heels! So whether you are heading to the beach with your girlfriends, need a quick style for work or are going out on a date, these styles will get you out the door without an ounce of stress.

In the chapters that follow I have created tutorials that will teach you how to create the five-minute hairstyle of your choice in five easy steps. There is also a glossary for you to look up any terms you're not familiar with. I've also included a few well-known favourites, to which I've added a touch of modern flair! But remember, what makes these looks so great is that there is plenty of room to add your own personal touch. Whether it's adjusting the style of plait you use, or adding a special accessory, you can make each of these styles your own – just focus on whatever looks good on you. So, follow the steps, get a feel for the possibilities and then let your imagination run wild.

Happy styling!

Jenny Strebe

Double twists into simple plait, pages 116-117

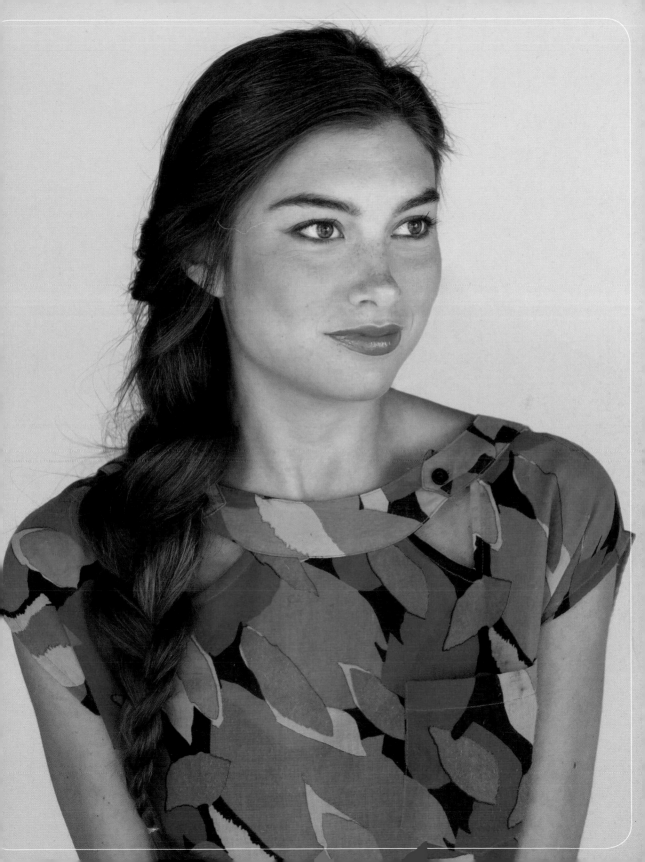

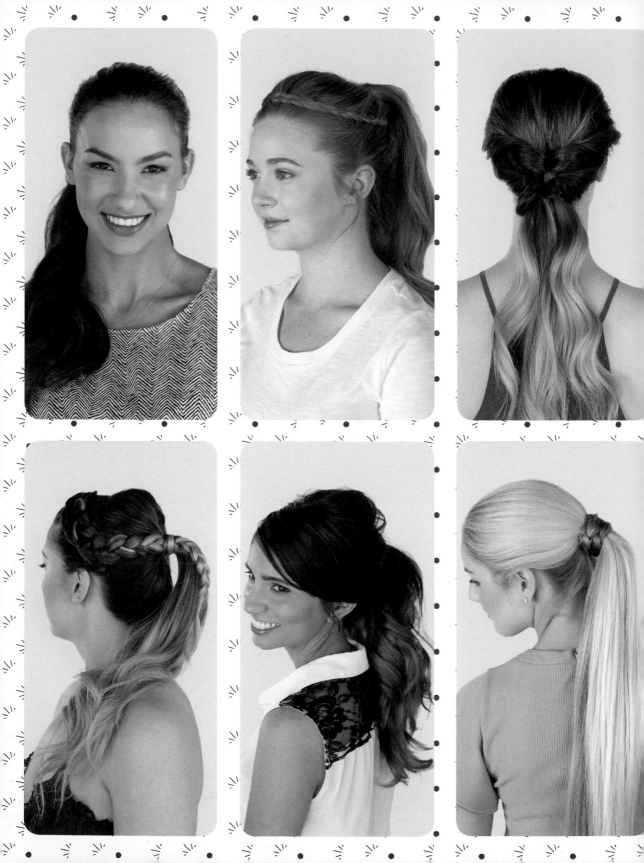

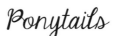

Ponytails

PLAITED-HEADBAND PONY

Whether you're sporty, girly or just need a little something extra to add to your everyday ponytail, the plaited headband pony is a great quick fix! While ideal on mid-length to long hair, this look is doable on short hair with just a few more grips. You can also go from day to night by curling your ponytail and adding some shine spray. All you need is a couple of hair bands, a comb and a hair grip.

1. Separate out a 5–8cm (2–3in) section of hair from behind one ear.

2. Divide this into three equal strands, then create a basic three-strand plait, taking the right strand over the middle, then taking the left strand over the new middle strand (originally the right strand) and so on.

3. Secure the end of the plait with a hair band. (You can also create fullness in your plait at this point by pulling on each section, as if you are fanning out a deck of cards.)

4. Bring the plait across the top of your head but do not pin it in place. Comb the rest of your hair back into a high ponytail.

5. Now hide the ends of the plait and the hair band by tucking them through the side of the ponytail, and securing them with a grip.

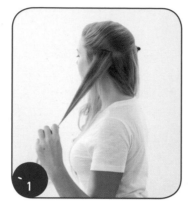

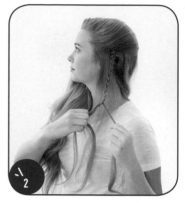

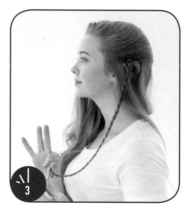

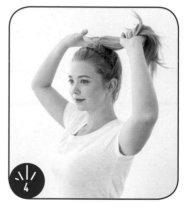

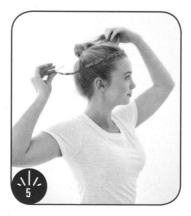

tip

If you have trouble keeping the base of your plait nice and tight at the roots, simply direct the sectioned-off hair upwards and plait in that direction.

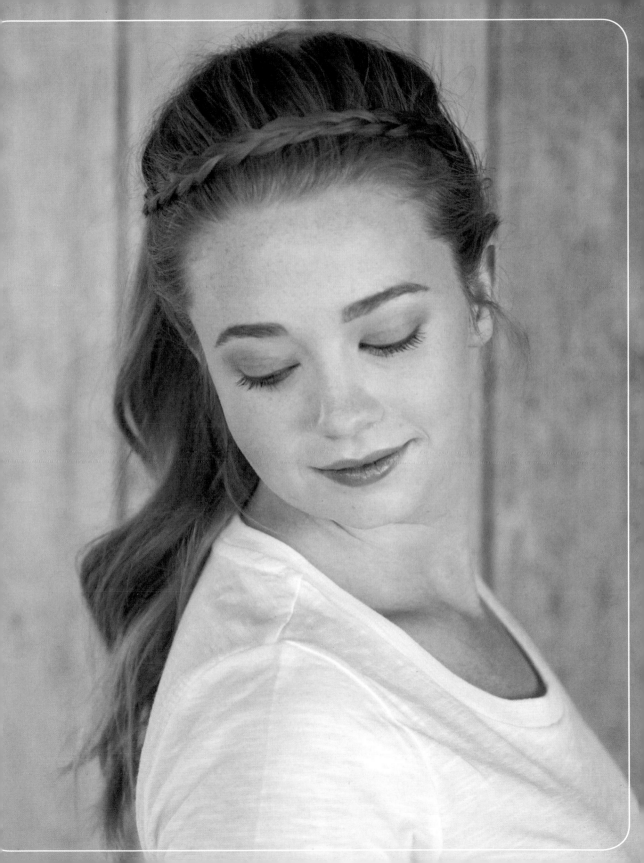

BOUFFANT PONY

This is a classic style with a modern twist. You can make this look as messy or as neat as you want, and in hardly any time at all. To make the ponytail more decorative, take a small section of hair (about 2.5cm/1in) from the ponytail and wrap it around the hair band. You can even plait the section before wrapping it if you want! All you'll need is a hair clip, a comb, a hair band and possibly a hair grip.

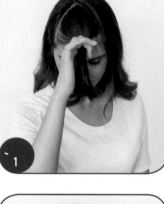

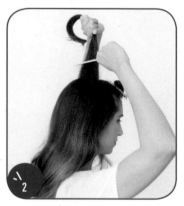

1. Part out a triangular section of hair from above your brow arch and clip it away for later.

2. Now take horizontal sections of hair from behind this triangular section and aggressively backcomb each one until you reach where your head begins to curve down towards your nape.

3. Now drop the backcombed hair and lightly comb over the top of it to create a sleeker look on the surface.

4. Gather all of your hair (apart from the triangular section) to the back of your head and secure it with a hair band.

5. Finally, unclip the triangular section and swoop it over to the side as desired, tucking it behind your ear, and using a grip to secure it if necessary.

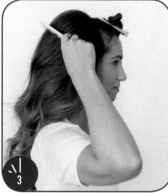

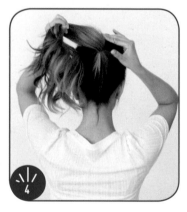

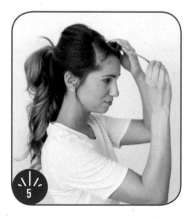

tip

When securing your ponytail with the hair band, be careful not to pull too tightly or you will lose volume in your bouffant.

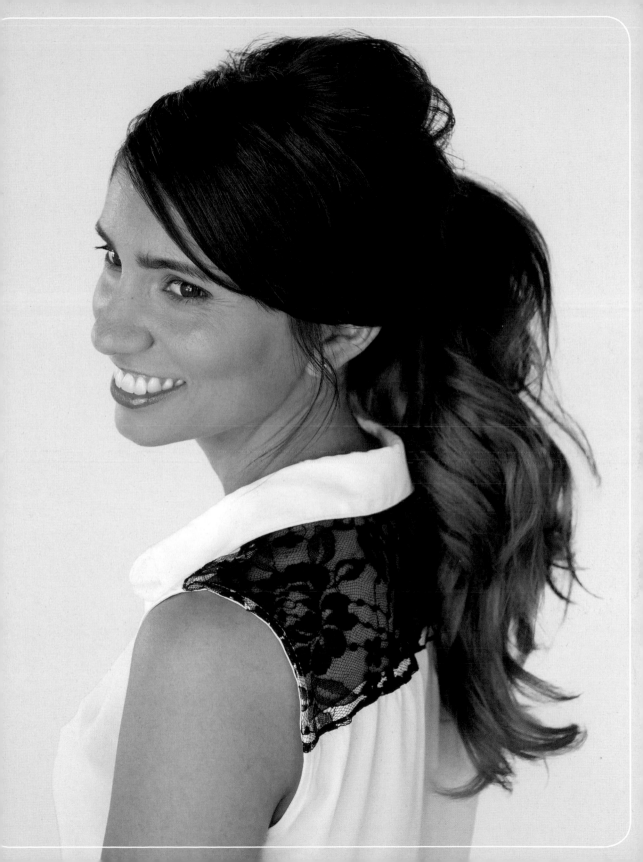

FAKE LONG PONY

Fake the look of long and luscious locks easily with this five-minute hairstyle! You'll find that there are no limits to the occasions when you can wear this pony, and you can make it even more your own simply by adding accessories or curls. For this simpler version, you will need nothing more than a comb, some hair clips and a couple of hair bands to complete the look.

1. Take a horseshoe-shaped section from your low crown to the bottom of your ear on either side and tie or clip the top sections out of the way for now.

2. Now use a hair band to secure the lower section of hair into a low ponytail.

3. Next, release the top sections of hair and create a second ponytail around 10cm (4in) above your first pony.

4. Lightly backcomb the base of both ponytails to create a fuller look.

5. To finish off, hold on to the base of the top ponytail and lightly pinch and pull the hair around your hairline to create a bit of extra fullness.

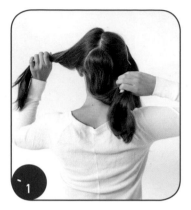

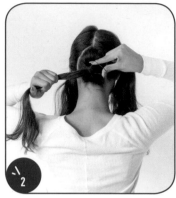

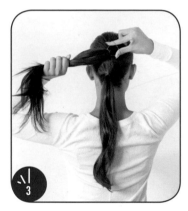

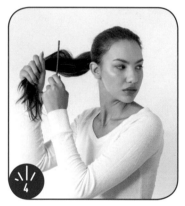

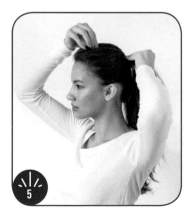

tip

This look works best on textured hair, since this will hide the bottom ponytail more effectively.

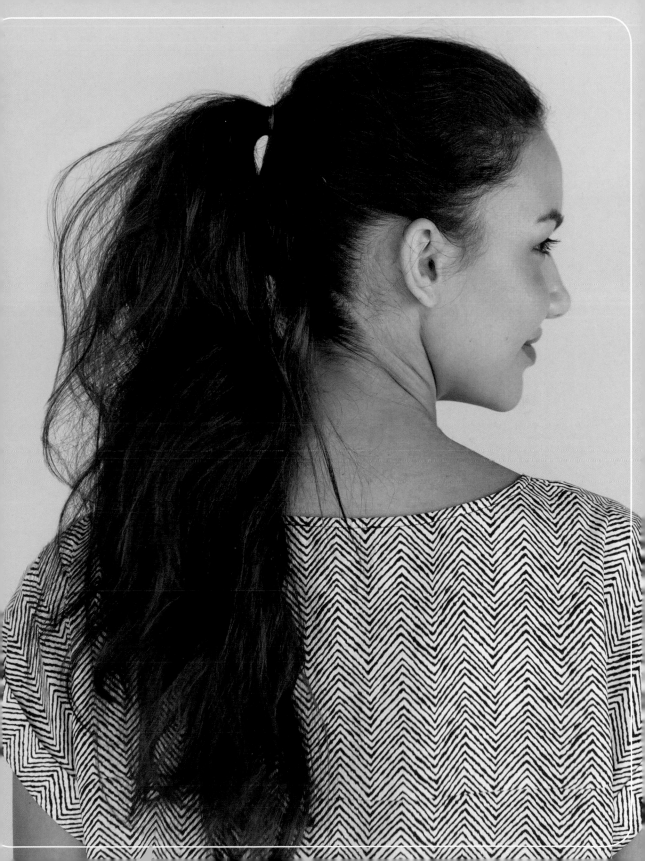

PLAIT INTO PONY

This is a great style for those of you who have a fringe you want to keep it out of your face. This look works for everyone, though – fringe or no fringe! It is quick to achieve with just a comb and two hair bands, and it lasts all day long, making it perfect for yoga, or for every day. You can also mix things up by trying a half-up half-down version (see the half-up rope-plait top knot on pages 64–65).

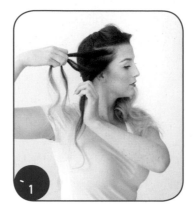

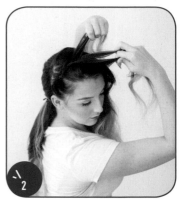

1. Divide your hair in half, separating the front from the back. Take a small section of hair from in front of one ear and divide this into three.

2. Start a 'lace plait' with these sections (working the strands underhand rather than the usual overhand), feeding portions of hair into the strands on either side of the plait as you progress.

3. Continue your plait, working right to left until you reach your opposite ear. Then continue with a regular plait until you reach the ends.

4. Secure this with a hair band, then 'pancake' your plait (pulling at sections of it) for fullness and texture.

5. Now pull all of your hair back into a high ponytail, incorporating the plait.

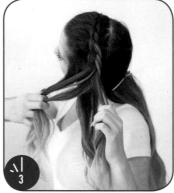

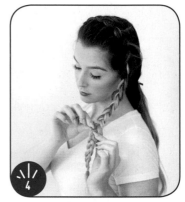

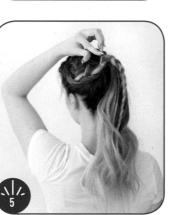

tip

For a fuller ponytail, start off by creating some waves or curls in your hair. You may also want to wrap a strand of hair around the hair band holding your pony (see right).

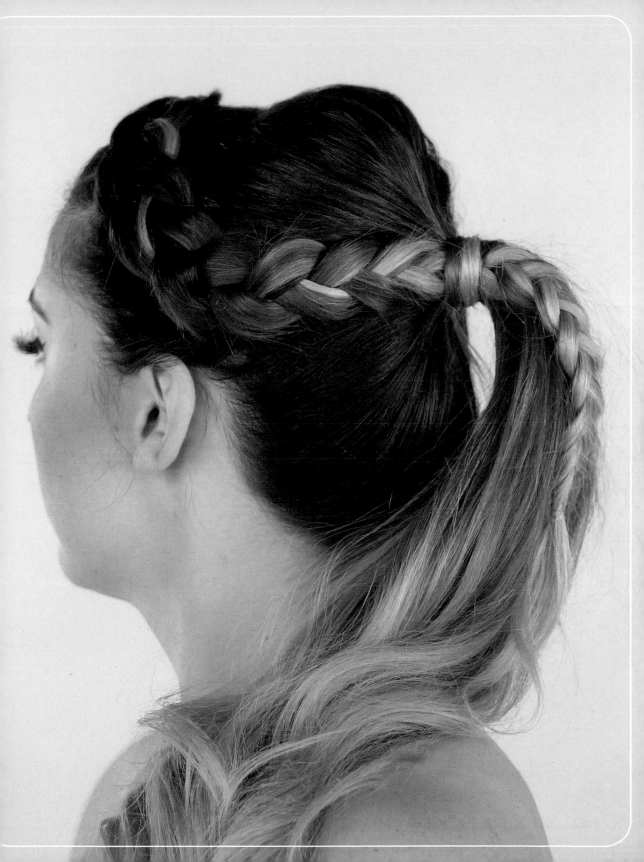

FULL FISHTAIL PONY

The full fishtail pony is a fun way to add volume and texture to your ponytail in just a few easy steps. The best thing about this hairstyle is that it looks great lived-in, so you don't have to worry about it getting a little messy throughout the day. Wear it from class to class, or at work all day. Grab two hair bands, a comb and some texturising spray and let's get started!

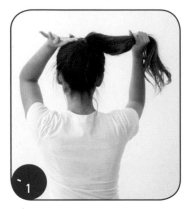

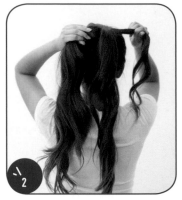

1. Create a high ponytail.

2. Divide this ponytail into two equal-sized sections. Now separate out a small strand of hair from the outside of the right section. This will pass up and over to become incorporated into the section of hair on the left. This action is then repeated on the left, with a small strand of hair taken from the far left, then passed up and over to join the right section. (See step 3 on page 36 for an additional view.)

3. Repeat until you reach your desired length of fishtail, then secure it with a hair band.

4. Apply some texturising spray, then pull at individual strands of the fishtail to create fullness.

5. For extra volume, grab the sides of the fishtail at the base of the ponytail and pull them outwards simultaneously.

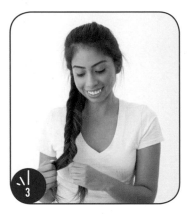

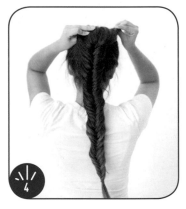

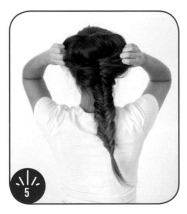

tip

If you want this style to have a high-ponytail effect, insert a few hair grips into the base of the ponytail.

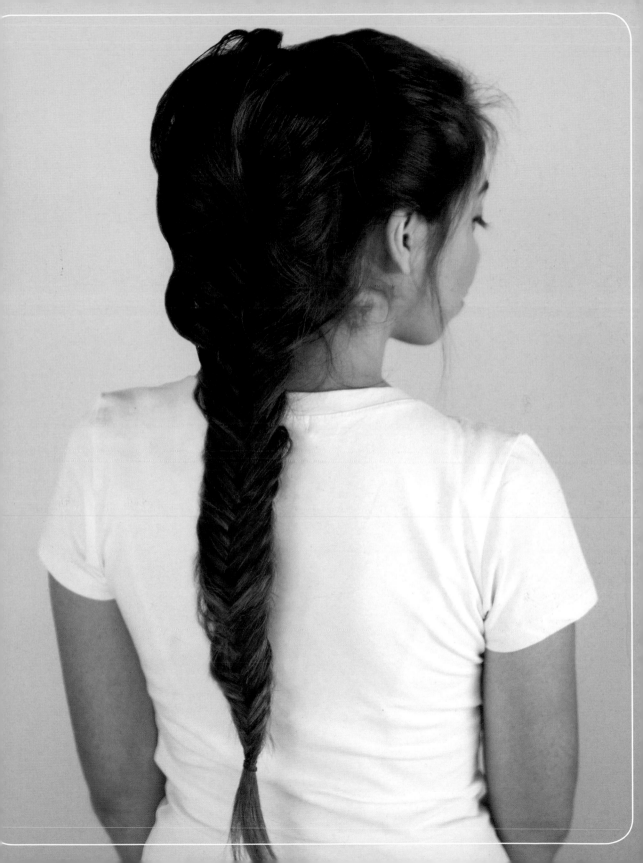

DOUBLE TOPSY-TAIL PONY

This is a modest and graceful hairstyle. It is incredibly easy to dress up or down, enabling you to create styles for all occasions, from errands to parties, using just two hair bands, a hair clip and a comb! If you would like more of a challenge, plait the ends of the top topsy-tail before pulling it through the bottom topsy-tail for some subtle texture.

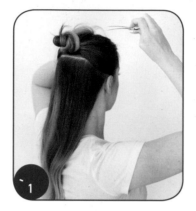

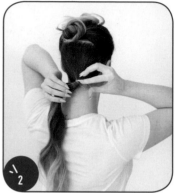

1. Divide your hair in half horizontally from ear to ear. Clip the top section out of the way for now.

2. Gather all the hair from the bottom section and, using a hair band, create a low ponytail at the nape of your neck.

3. Create a hole in the middle of the base of the ponytail, then pull your hair up and fold it back on itself, threading it down through this hole. This creates your topsy-tail.

4. Now release the top section and create a ponytail directly above the bottom ponytail. Then make a second topsy-tail to sit above the previous one.

5. Finally, feed the hair from your top topsy-tail down through the bottom topsy-tail to complete the look.

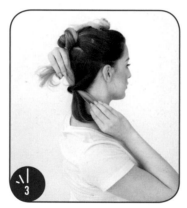

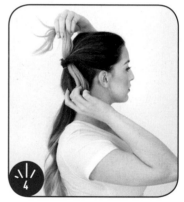

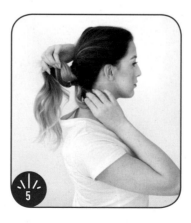

tip

To create a fuller effect, lightly spritz each topsy-tail with some texturising spray and then gently pull the strands outwards.

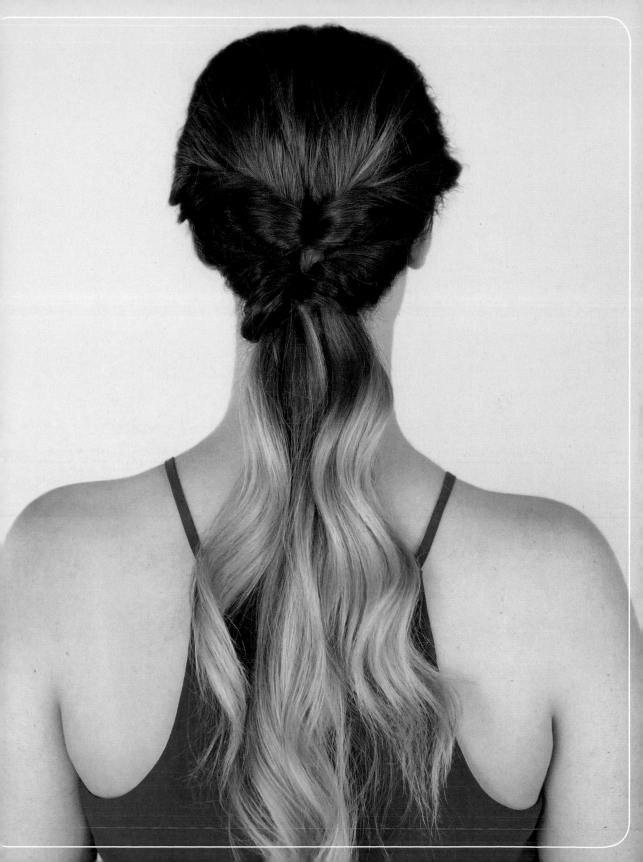

SLEEK WRAPPED PONY

The sleek wrapped pony is a classic wear-everywhere style, equally suited to dressed-up or casual looks. It is easiest to do on mid-length to long straight hair, but if your hair fits into a ponytail, then give it a try! A hair band, some serum, a hair grip and a comb are all you'll need. To make it fun and flirty, you can even plait the small section of hair first (as on page 24).

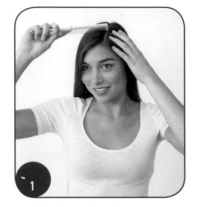

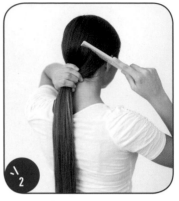

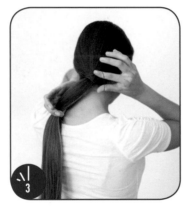

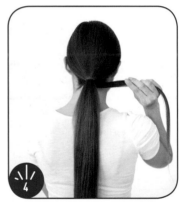

1. Part your hair neatly to the desired side.

2. Comb your hair and gather it tightly at the nape of your neck. Make sure there are no lumps or bumps, and use a bit of light serum to make sure you get rid of any flyaways.

3. Hold the base of the ponytail firmly and secure it with a hair band. To keep your ponytail central you can try keeping your head parallel to the floor.

4. Now separate out a 2.5cm (1in) section of hair from the ponytail on the underside.

5. Wrap this small section neatly around the hair band. To secure it in place, loop the end of the sectioned-out hair around a hair grip, and then push the grip under and into the base of the ponytail.

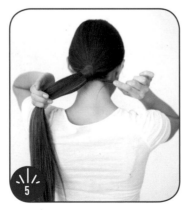

tip

If your hair is naturally curly, give it a sleeker look before you start. Towel-dry it, then blow-dry it straight down with a paddle brush.

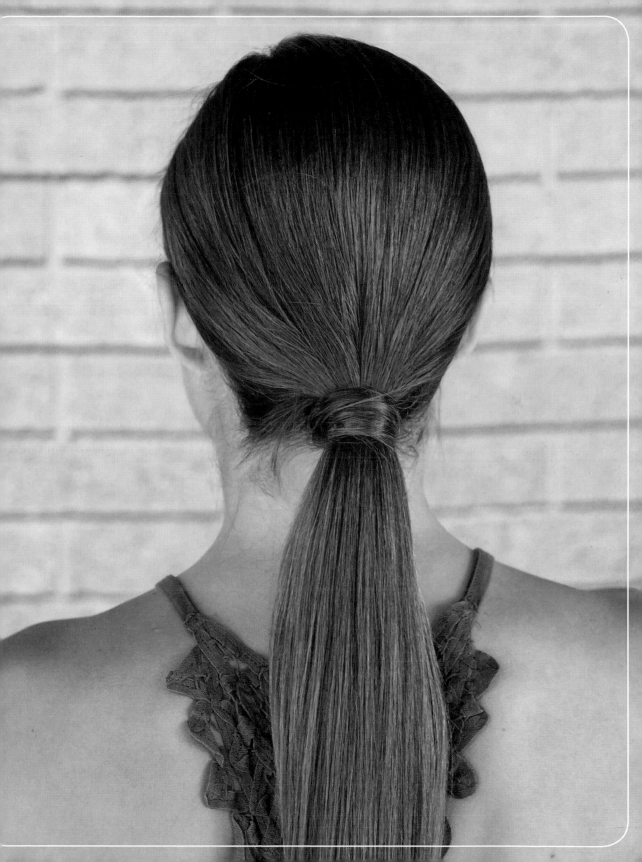

PLAIT-WRAPPED PONY

The plait-wrapped pony is a time-efficient style that's suitable for everyone. In just a few minutes you get a chic look with a flirty twist. This hairstyle can be worn casually or to a special event – it's completely adaptable. And the only items you'll need to achieve it are a comb, a hair band and a few hair grips.

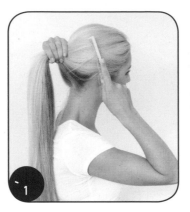

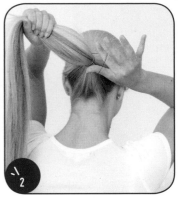

1. Comb through all of your hair, making sure there are no knots in it. Pull all of your hair to the lower back of your head.

2. Secure your hair in place here with a hair band.

3. Separate out a 2.5cm (1in) section from the ponytail on its underside, then clip the remainder of the ponytail out of the way for now.

4. Now create a simple plait with this small section of hair, and secure it with a hair band.

5. Unclip the rest of the ponytail and then wrap the plait around the base of the hair band. Secure it in place using a hair grip or two.

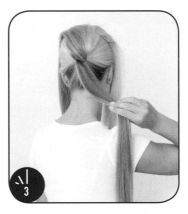

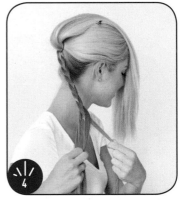

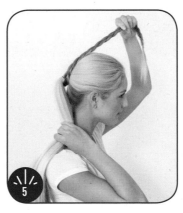

tip

If you have thin hair, pull and stretch out the sectioned-off plait before you wrap it around the hair band to create more fullness.

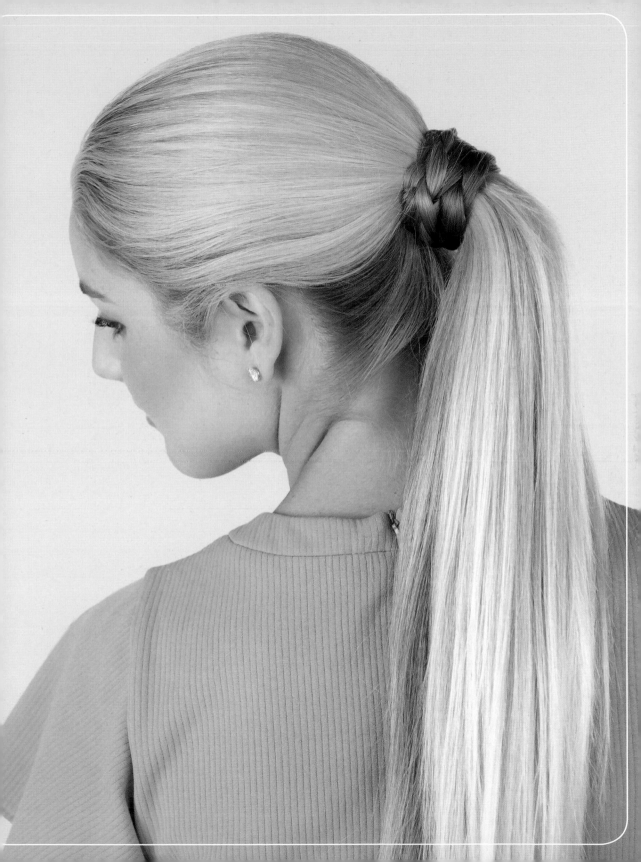

DOUBLE-PONY POUF

The double-pony pouf is a really quick and feminine hairstyle. It's perfect if you want to keep things simple. And, if you want to add a bit more texture and edge, you can always curl your hair prior to styling it. As with all of the styles in this book, the tools you'll need are minimal – a comb and a few hair bands. That's it!

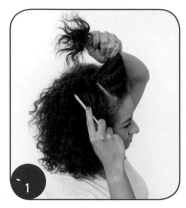

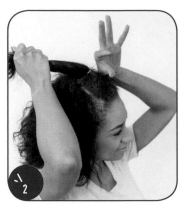

1. Separate out a small triangular section of hair from brow arch to brow arch, going back roughly 8–10cm (3–4in) from your hairline (depending on the density of your hair).

2. Create your first ponytail by securing this sectioned-out hair with a hair band.

3. While holding on to the base of the ponytail, pull the gathered strands forwards to create your first pouf.

4. Now gather up the rest of your hair and create another ponytail, securing it with a hair band.

5. Hold on to the base of this second ponytail and pinch and pull the strands out as before to create volume and fullness with this second pouf.

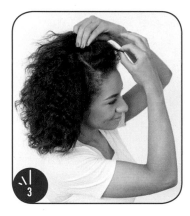

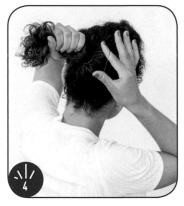

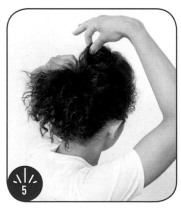

tip

If your hair lacks volume and texture, you may find it helpful to backcomb both of your poufs prior to securing them with hair bands.

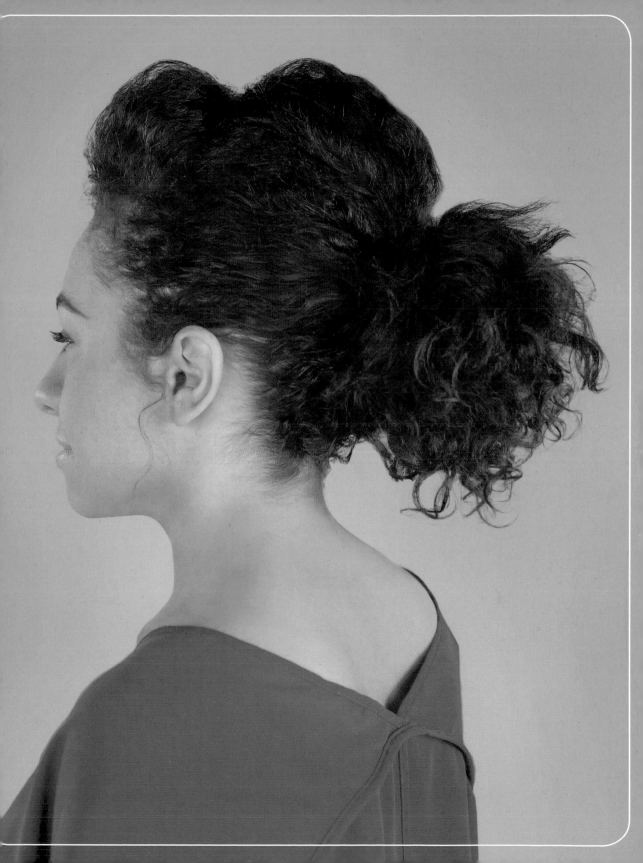

TEXTURED PONY

This quick, cute hairstyle is great for everyday use, and you don't even need a comb – using your fingers to comb through your hair instead will help to create more natural texture. You can use your fingers to backcomb out the ponytail, too, if you want to create a little more volume and drama. Just grab a hair band and some curling tongs and you'll be ready to start.

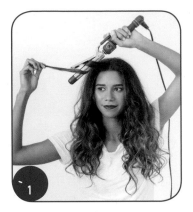

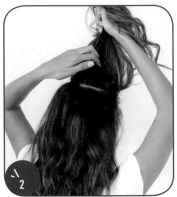

1. Start by adding some curls and texture to your hair by wrapping 2.5–5cm (1–2in) sections of hair around your curling iron. Just a few strands here and there will be enough, although if you have time on your hands you can go as far as you like!

2. Next take small sections of hair and lightly backcomb them at the roots with your fingers.

3. Now gently comb your hair back with your fingers. It's very important not to lose any texture or volume while you are doing this.

4. Create a high ponytail by gathering your hair towards the high-crown area, securing it with a hair band.

5. Finally, pinch and pull at your roots to create a bit more volume. Hold on to your ponytail while you do this so that you don't dislodge it.

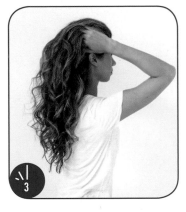

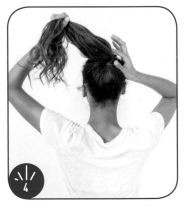

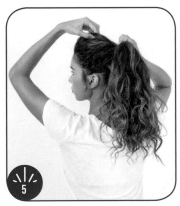

tip

If you want to mix this style up in a hurry, try playing with different textures by adding more curls or a plait.

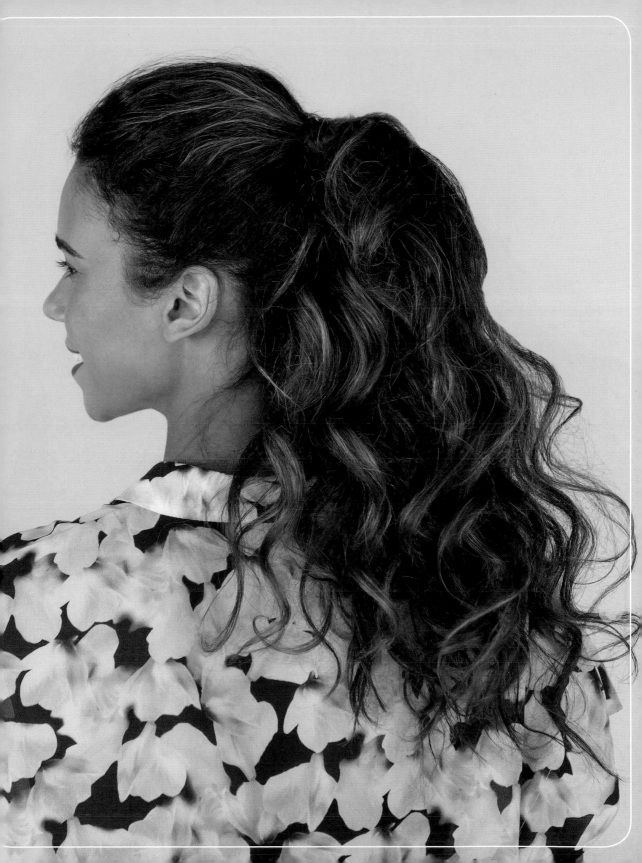

FAUX-HAWK PONY

The faux-hawk pony offers you a great party style in a pinch. Created with a simple pulled-out Dutch plait feeding into a ponytail, this style will give you an edgy look in under five minutes! What's more, you can wear this look all night long without worrying about maintenance, since it still looks amazing when it's lived-in. All you need is a comb, a hair clip and two hair bands.

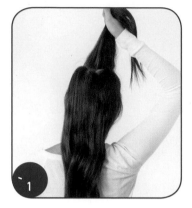
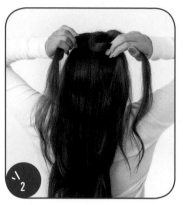
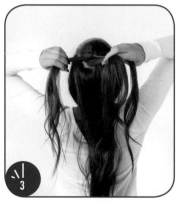
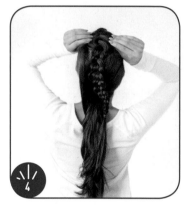

1. Separate out a triangular section of hair at your forehead. (Clip the rest of your hair out of the way, if it helps.)

2. Grab a 2.5–5cm (1–2in) section at the top of the triangle and divide it in three for your plait.

3. Unlike the inverted look of a French plait, a Dutch plait sits above the hair – each side strand passes under the middle strand and then up (the reverse of the French over-and-down movement). Start plaiting the triangular section, absorbing new strands of hair from either side, as for a French plait.

4. Continue with a regular plait for a little way beyond the triangular section, secure it with a hair band, then stretch out your plait for the faux-hawk effect.

5. Gather everything up into a single ponytail.

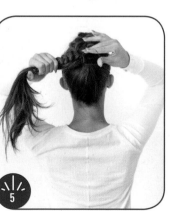

tip

If you want to create an even larger faux-hawk effect, backcomb the hair in your triangular section prior to plaiting it.

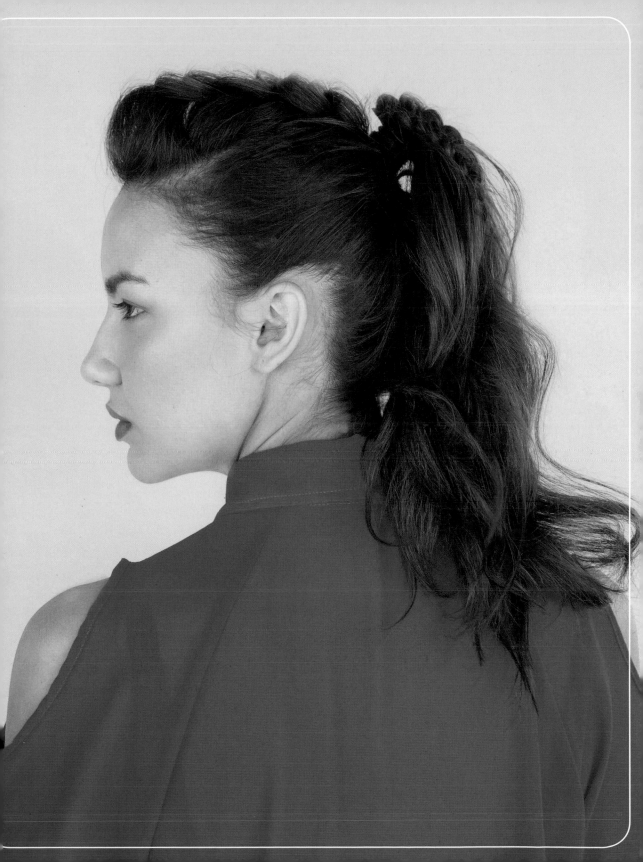

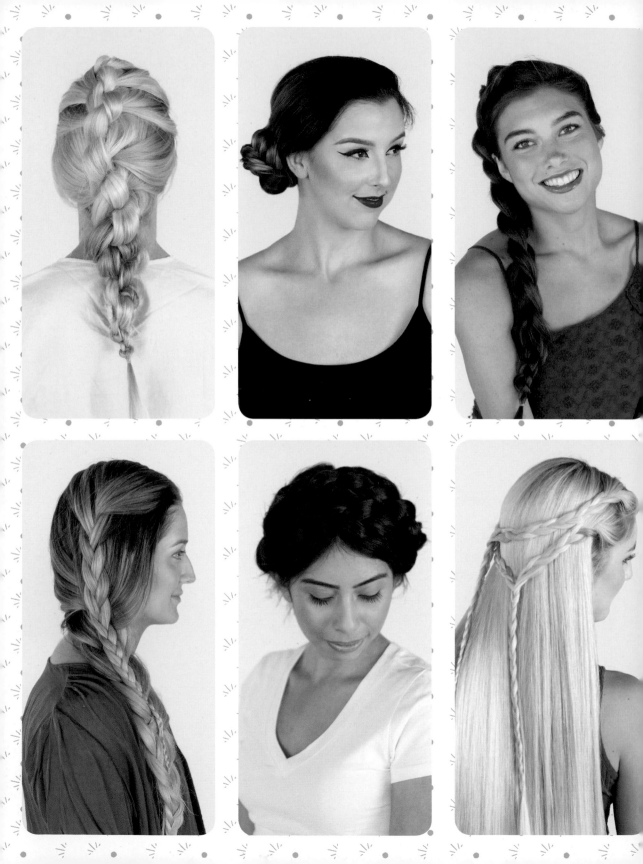

2

Plaits

KNOTTED FRENCH PLAIT

The knotted French plait is a beautiful style that works well with both classic and more edgy looks, and it is very easy to adapt for all sorts of events. If your hair is straight, you can leave it as it is, or you can add curls. If your hair is short, you can adapt the knotted French plait and make it a bun instead. Just grab a comb and a hair band, and let's get started.

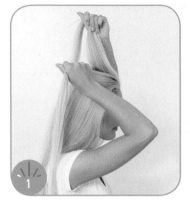

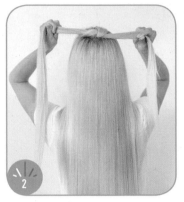

1. Starting from your hairline above your forehead, separate out a section of hair (roughly 5–8cm/2–3in) and then divide this section in two.

2. Cross one section over the other, then loop it under and through to create a knot. Pull both sides firmly to tighten the knot.

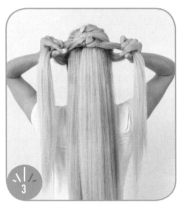

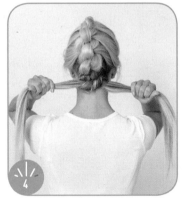

3. Now take two more sections from the hairline of your face and level with the top of your knot, and incorporate them into each of the strands emerging from the first knot. Now tie another knot.

4. Continue this process until you reach the nape of your neck, then tie knots with the remaining two strands to your desired length and secure the ends with a hair band.

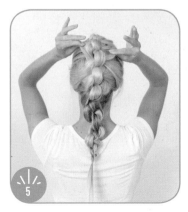

5. Finish off by stretching and pulling the knots to create volume and texture.

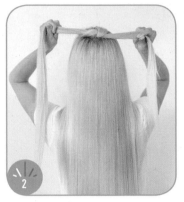

tip

Silky hair can be prone to slipping out of the knots. Try adding texture before styling by applying mousse or sea-salt spray to damp hair and then blow-drying it.

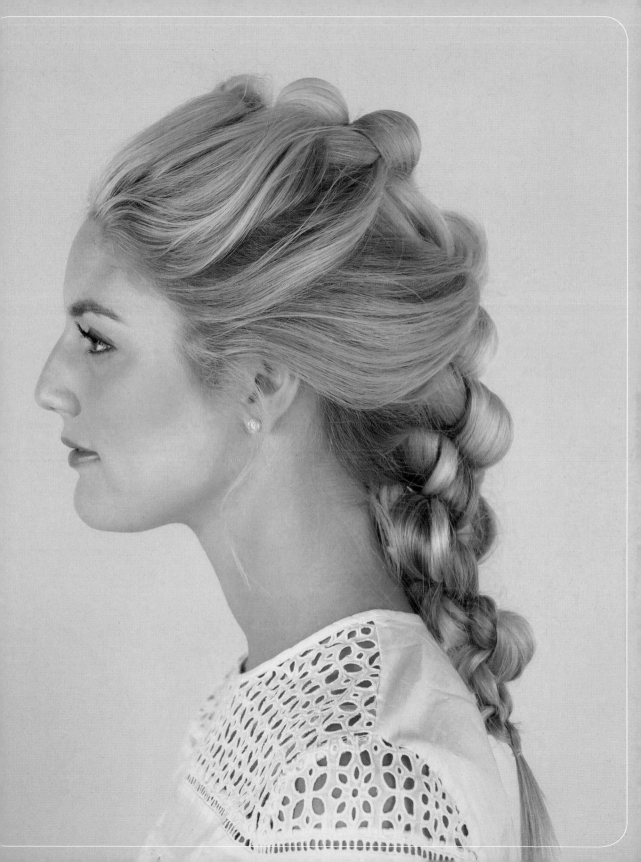

SIDE FISHTAIL BUN

The side fishtail bun is a trendy spin on your everyday side bun. It's fun, flirty and easier to do than you think. This hairstyle is perfect for second-day hair; texture is definitely your friend for this look! Wear it for a special occasion or out to lunch with friends. Before you begin, gather together a hair band, comb, hair grips and some hairspray.

1. Gather all of your hair to the desired side, and create a ponytail by securing it with a hair band.

2. Divide your ponytail into two equal sections.

3. Take a small piece of hair from the far side of the right section of the ponytail and add it to the left section, then repeat with the other side. Continue crisscrossing in this way until you've created your fishtail, then secure the ends with a hair band.

4. Now wrap your fishtail plait around the hair band to create the bun and secure it in place with hair grips.

5. To finish, gently pull at random tiny sections of hair from the crown of your head, to give the style some softness.

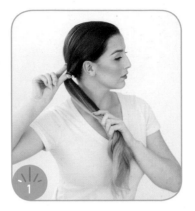

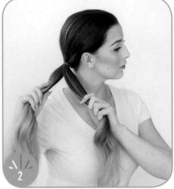

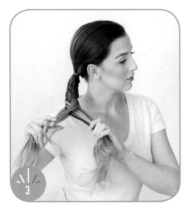

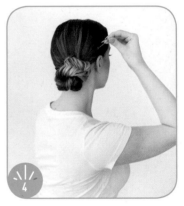

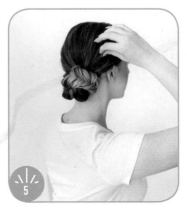

tip

If your hair is fine, pulling and stretching the fishtail plait prior to creating your bun will give you a much fuller effect.

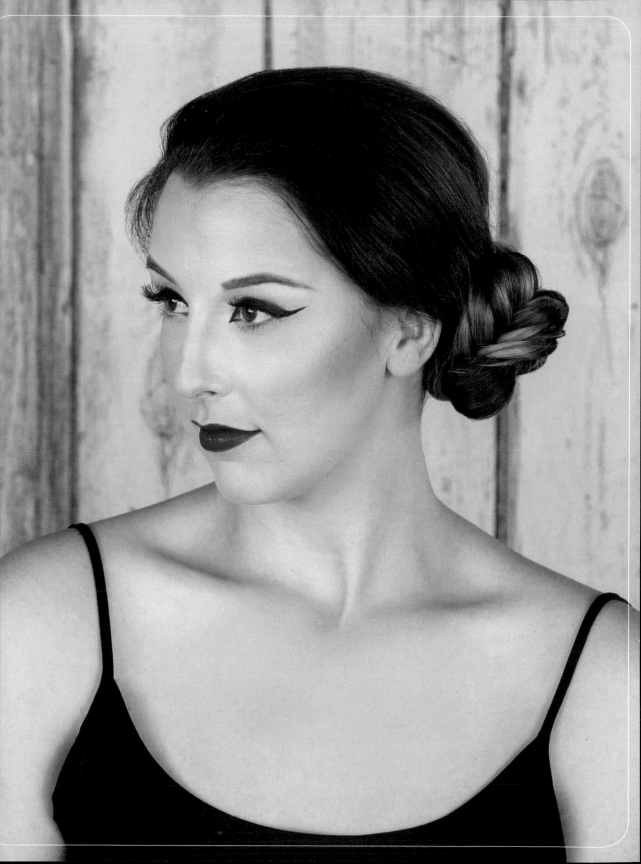

SIDE ROPE PLAIT

If you've ever twirled or twisted your hair, then you know how to create a rope plait! It may look tricky, but it is actually one of the easiest styles in this book. It is a quick, elegant way to get that second-day hair out of your face, and requires nothing more than a comb and a hair band. If you don't want your plait to the side, then create it at the back, or throw it up into a ponytail.

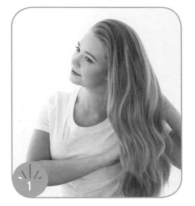

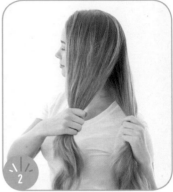

1. Start with 'textured' hair (hair that hasn't been washed for a day or so is perfect!). Pull your hair over to the desired side.

2. Divide your hair into two equal sections. Take the section to the front and start twisting it clockwise (towards your face).

3. Now take that section up and over the back section. Your front section should now be at the back. Now twist the second section clockwise.

4. Pass this newly twisted section up over the other section, then continue this up-and-over process until you reach your desired length of plait. Secure it with a hair band.

5. To give your plait some extra volume and a lived-in look, lightly pinch and pull pieces out of both twisted portions.

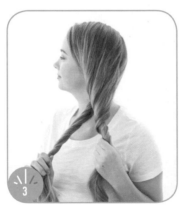

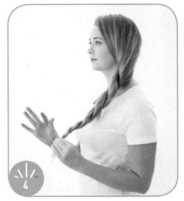

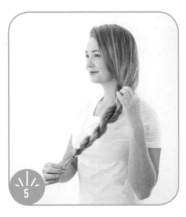

tip

If your hair is extremely layered and prone to falling out of place, curl your hair first. Curls will blend in better with the rope plait.

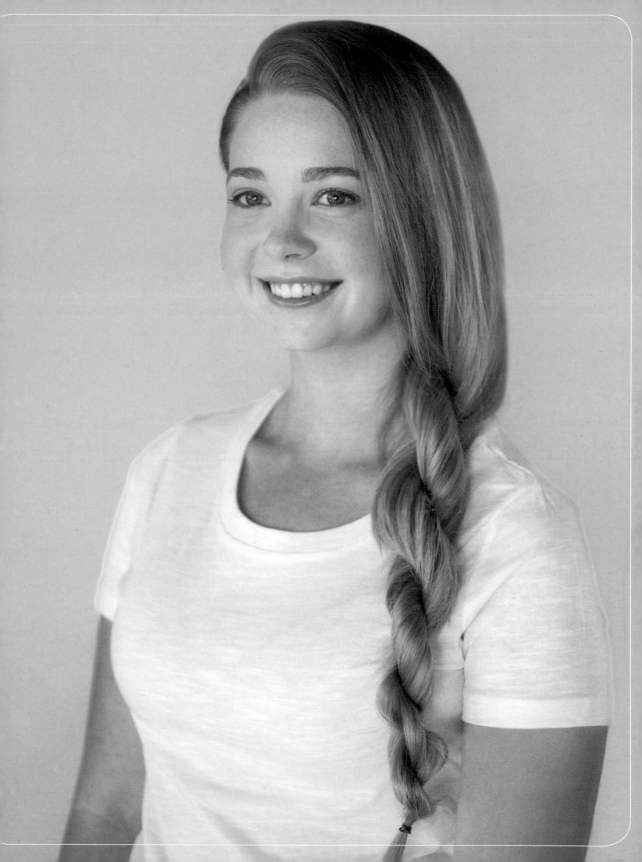

TUXEDO PLAIT

This is the deluxe version of a standard half-up half-down style! Taking the extra step is simple but looks like you've made a whole lot of effort, and who doesn't love a hairstyle that looks harder than it is? Two hair bands and a comb are all that you'll need, plus some texturising spray if your hair is slippery. If you're a little more plait-savvy, you can try substituting a fishtail plait (see pages 18–19).

1. Separate out a large section of hair on top of your head using a horseshoe-shaped parting.

2. Divide this horseshoe section into three strands and use them to create a simple plait. Plait right down and secure the ends with a hair band.

3. Now 'pancake' out the plait to make it fuller. Apply a texturising spray if your hair is prone to slipping out of place.

4. Next, take a small strand of hair from in front of each ear but below the horseshoe section.

5. Take both of these sections and criss-cross them over the plait. Then, holding the end of the plait up out of the way, connect the two sections with a hair band that will then be hidden underneath the hanging plait.

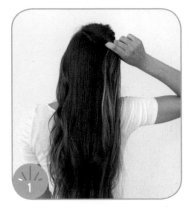

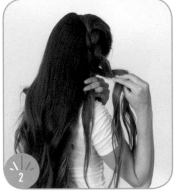

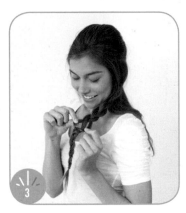

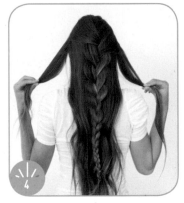

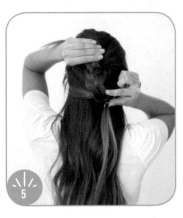

tip

If you want your hair to look fuller and longer, simply attach a few hair extensions for a more dramatic look.

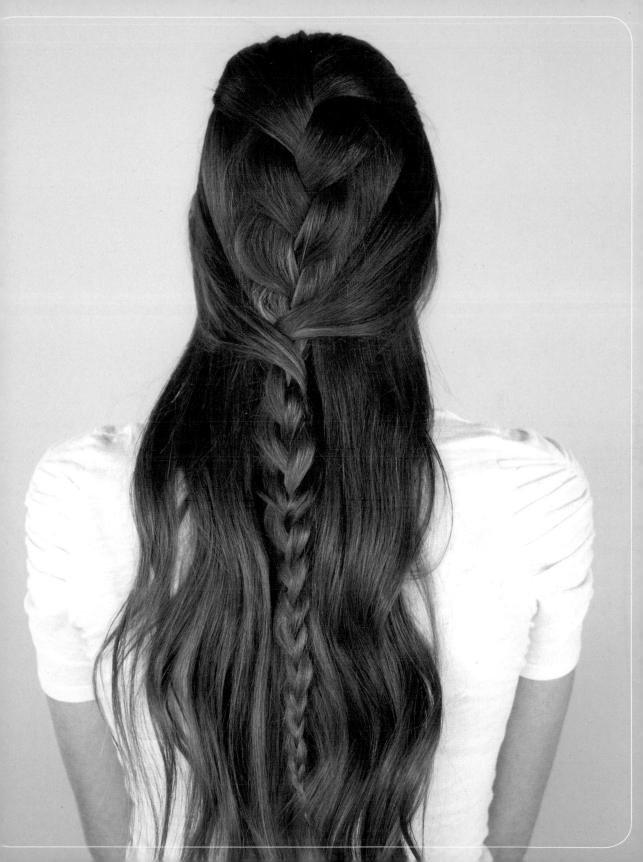

STACKED SIDE PLAIT

This quick tutorial offers a handy way to make your everyday side plait look more intricate. All you do is create two plaits and then intertwine them with the help of a comb, a few hair bands and some hair grips. This will result in a look that will take you effortlessly from poolside to happy hour out with your friends.

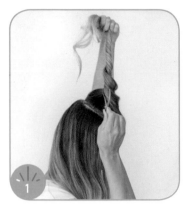 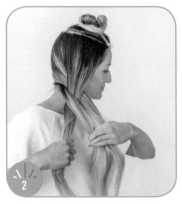

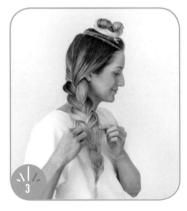 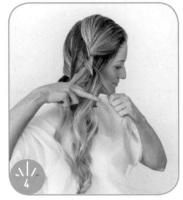

1. Divide your hair into two sections horizontally, with the bottom section denser than the top. Clip away the top section for later.

2. With the bottom section, create a standard plait on your desired side.

3. Secure the end of the plait with a hair band, then 'pancake' the plait to create more volume and texture.

4. Now release the top section of hair and use it to create a tight plait right over the top of the lower plait. Secure the ends with another hair band.

5. Connect the top plait to the bottom plait by taking the end of the top plait and looping it through the bottom plait. Secure the two plaits together with a hair grip on the underside of the plaits.

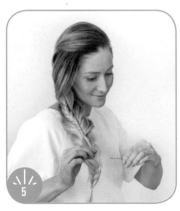

tip

If you fancy a looser, more feminine look, try leaving some strands of hair out of the plaits and curling them.

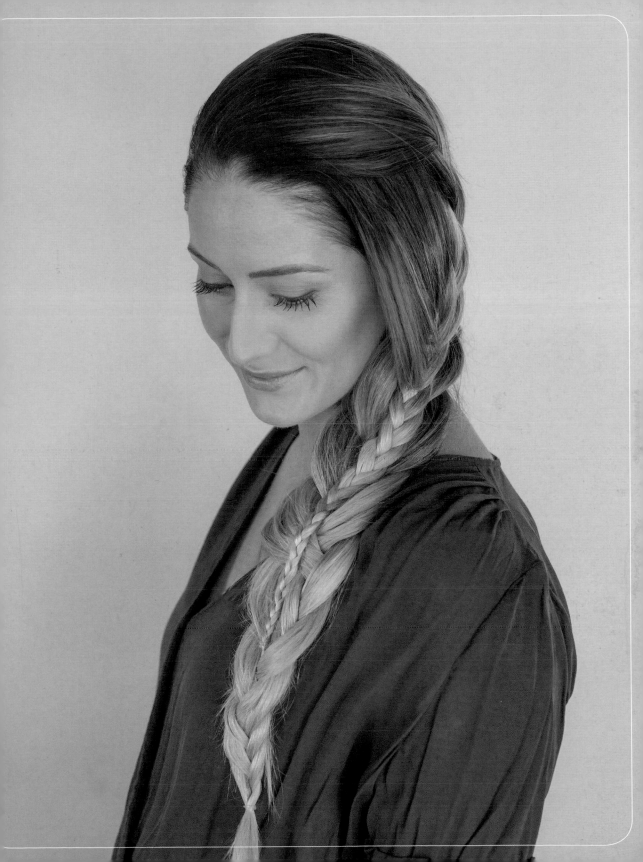

TWIN-PLAIT HALF-DOWN

This super-quick style is great for longer hair, and you'll need nothing more than a comb, a hair clip and some hair bands to complete it. The plaits come together to create a classic and delicate look that you can then play around with, depending on your mood. Wear this versatile look anywhere and embrace the compliments that will come your way!

1. Part your hair to the desired side. Take a triangular section of hair, around 5–8cm (2–3in) wide, from the right side of your head and create a plait. Once you are halfway down, clip the plait away for later, then repeat on the other side.

2. Take both plaits to the back of your head and overdirect them towards your left side. Clip both plaits together.

3. Now connect the plaits by incorporating them both into a new plait. Secure the ends with a hair band.

4. Clip this first finished plait out of the way.

5. Now repeat steps 1 to 3, this time using sections taken from underneath the top plait and directed to the right instead of the left. Unclip the top section and place it over the bottom plait to finish.

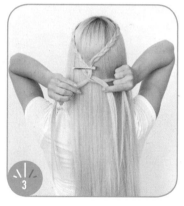
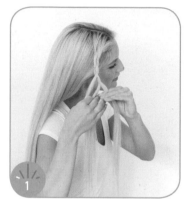
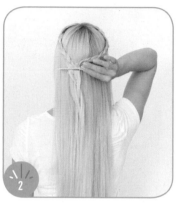
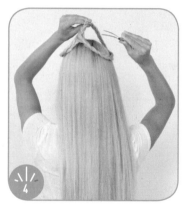
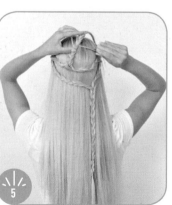

tip

If you would like a longer plait, simply adding in some hair extensions before styling will give you an instant solution!

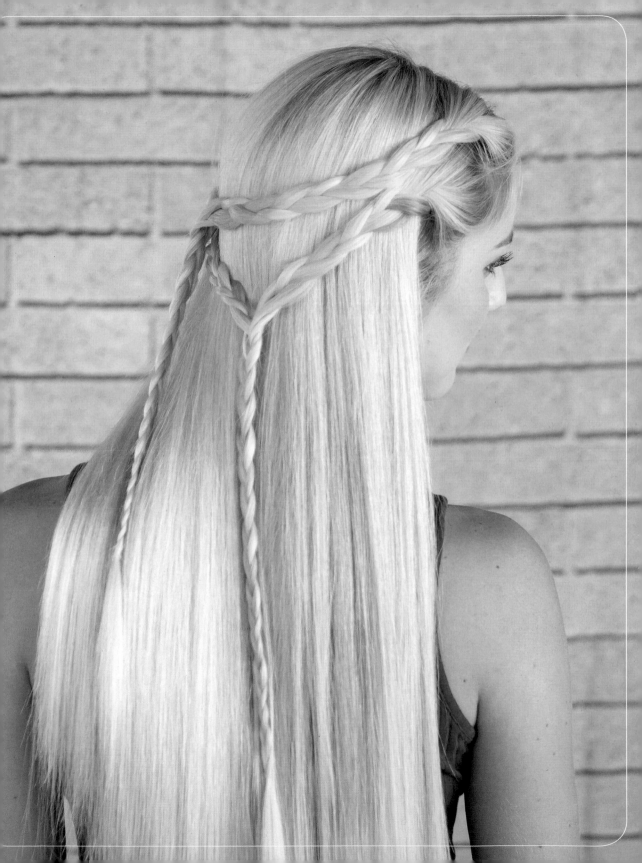

MILKMAID PLAIT

This is the new messy bun – simple, stylish and perfect for pool parties or hanging out with girlfriends. You can wear it effortlessly all day long, and the bonus is that it makes for great second-day hair once you take the plaits out. It's best on long, unlayered hair, but if you have shorter hair, try a half-up half-down version. Grab a comb, a couple of hair bands and some hair grips and let's begin!

1. Divide your hair vertically into two equal sections.

2. Starting on the right side, create a simple plait, securing the end with a hair band, and then do the same on the left side of your head.

3. Take each plait and gently 'pancake' each segment out. This will give your plaits a fuller appearance.

4. Now take the right plait and drape it over the top of your head. Then do the same with the left plait.

5. Finally, use as many hair grips as you need to secure both plaits in place.

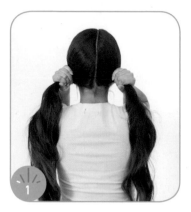

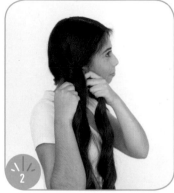

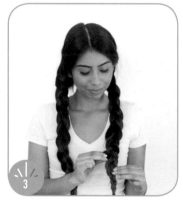

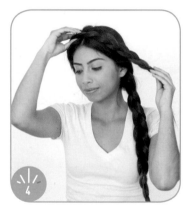

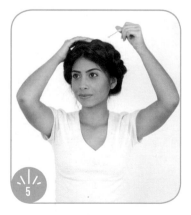

tip

To make this look a little more formal, use a shine spray to get rid of any flyaways.

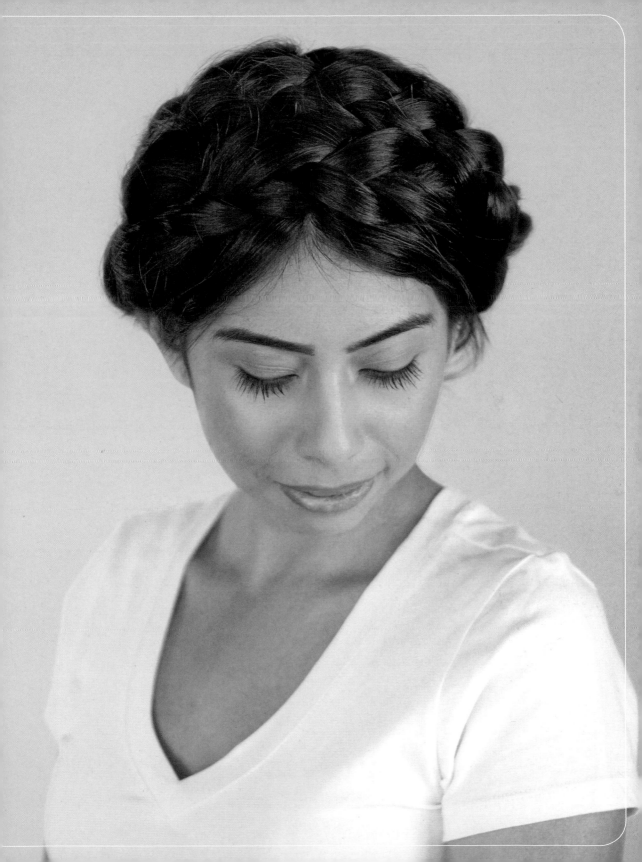

BOXER PLAITS

Boxer plaits are a great go-to look – they're perfect for keeping your hair out of your eyes at the gym, and then just as perfect for lunch with your girlfriends afterwards. You can style this look on clean hair or second-day hair. Either way, this 'do is achieved in just a few minutes, and it will see you right through the day. Throw a comb and two hair bands in your gym bag and you'll be set!

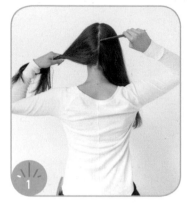
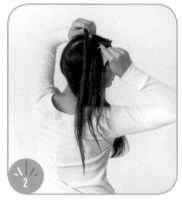

1. Divide your hair evenly in half down the centre, then comb through it.

2. On the right side, separate out a triangular section at your hairline and divide it into three equal strands.

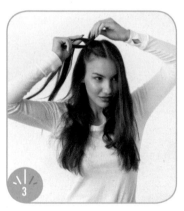
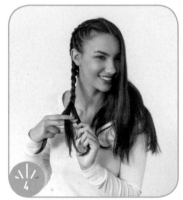

3. Begin your first plait by taking the right strand under and into the middle, then take the left strand under and into the middle. This reversal of the French-plait method will produce a Dutch plait, which sits out from the head. Incorporate hair into your sections as you progress.

4. When you reach the nape of your neck, continue with a regular Dutch plait until you reach the ends, then secure them with a hair band.

5. Repeat for the left-hand plait.

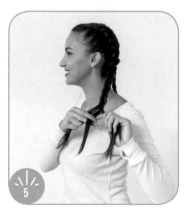

tip

If your hair is prone to flyaways then dampen it prior to starting. This will also help to create tighter plaits.

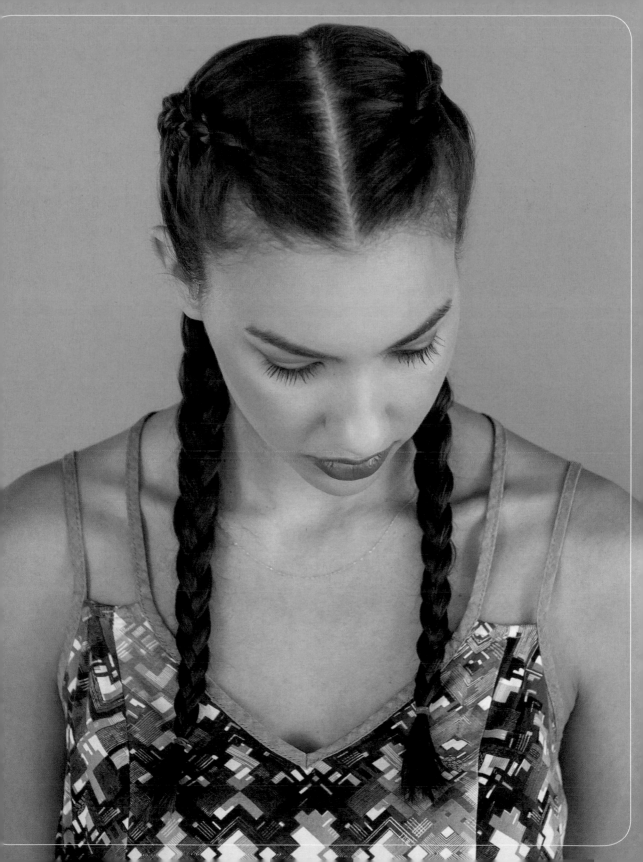

DUTCH SIDE PLAIT

As mentioned earlier, a Dutch plait is very similar to a French plait in terms of technique, but with the Dutch plait sitting above the hair, it is a lot easier to make this style your own. Add volume by pulling on the strands of the plait, or add texture by backcombing your roots before plaiting. This style is ideal for long and medium-thick hair. Have a hair band and a comb ready before starting!

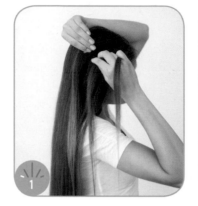

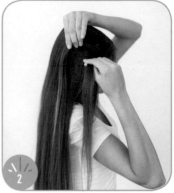

1. Part your hair to the desired side. Take a section from the top and then divide it into three strands.

2. Start your plait by taking the right strand under and into the middle, then taking your left section under and into the middle.

3. Now begin feeding small sections of hair into the plait. Incorporate a 2.5cm (1in) section into the left strand and bring it under and into the middle. Then do the same with the right strand, and so on.

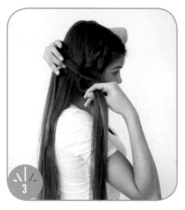

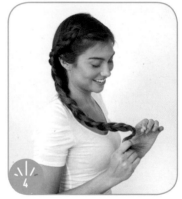

4. When all your hair has been incorporated, continue plaiting to the end of your hair, and tie it with a hair band.

5. 'Pancake' the individual strands to create a fuller-looking plait.

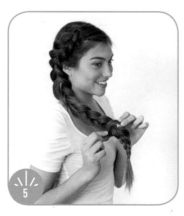

tip

If your hair is fine and you want a fatter plait, try blow-drying your hair with a texturising or sea-salt spray prior to plaiting.

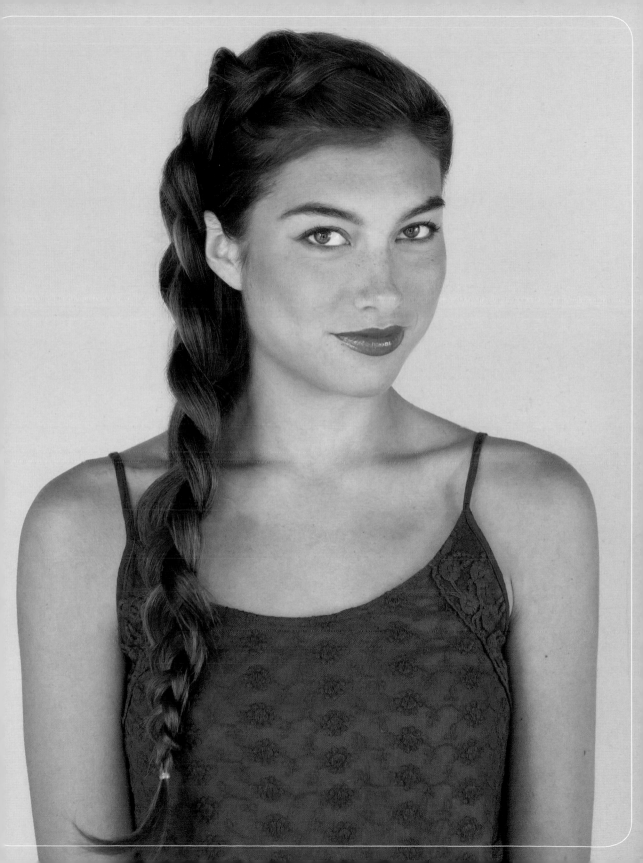

LOW ROPE PLAIT

Why not try giving your everyday plait a twist with this quick alternative? You can wear this versatile hairdo anywhere – to work or to the beach – and it has the bonus of highlighting any contrasting tones in your hair. The best part? Keep it clean or a little messy – either looks great! You'll need nothing more than a comb and two hair bands to create it.

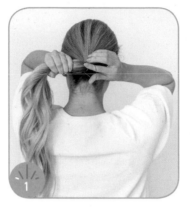 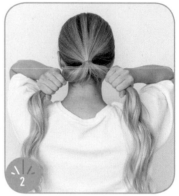

1. Comb your hair to your low nape and secure it in place with a hair band.

2. Now divide the hair of the ponytail into two equal strands.

3. Begin by twisting the right strand in a clockwise direction a few times.

4. Now take the twisted right strand up and over the left so that the left strand is now on the right. Repeat the previous step, this time twisting the new right strand clockwise and taking it up and over the other strand. When twisting your two sections together you should be working in an anticlockwise direction.

5. Repeat this process until you've reached your desired length, then secure the ends of the plait with a hair band.

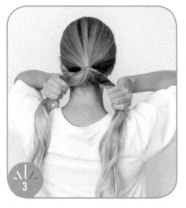 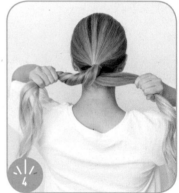

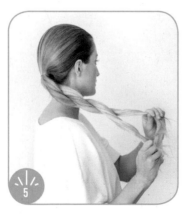

tip

You can easily make this look your own by changing the location of the rope plait, or by adding more texture.

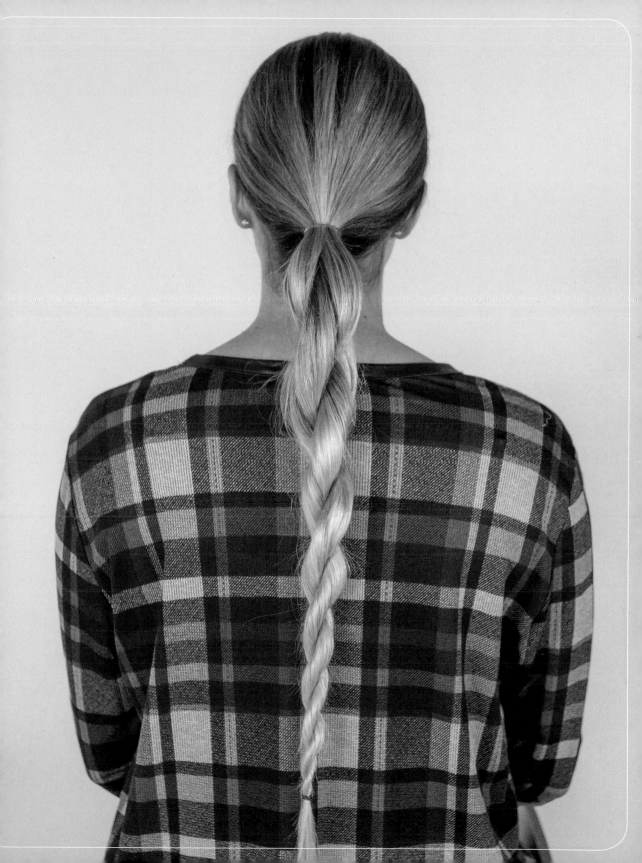

MERMAID-STYLE DOUBLE PLAIT

This hairstyle is great for those of you with long, thick hair. It's a beautiful look for a date or just hanging out with friends. And best of all, it looks much harder than it is! As with all of the styles in this book, all you need are everyday tools – a hair clip, a couple of hair bands, hair grips and a comb. You can also mix up the two different plaits to suit your own personal style.

1. Divide your hair in half horizontally; the top section should be a little smaller than the bottom. Clip the top section out of the way for now.

2. Create a simple three-strand plait with the bottom section and secure it with a hair band.

3. Now release the top section and use it to create a fishtail plait (see page 18). Secure it with another hair band.

4. Next, flip the top plait up out of the way, and 'pancake' the bottom plait by stretching the sections out aggressively. This will create extra volume.

5. To finish, tuck the end of the fishtail into the lower plait. To prevent the top plait from slipping out, lift both plaits and secure the end of the fishtail from behind by weaving a hair grip through from the back.

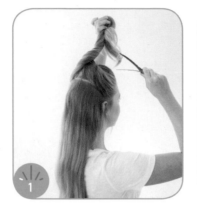

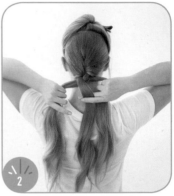

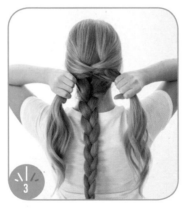

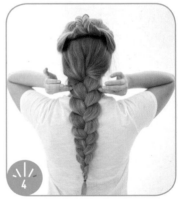

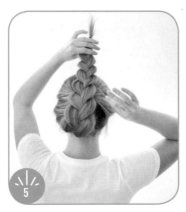

tip

If your hair is silky and prone to slipping out of plaits, simply apply a texturising spray or a dry shampoo before starting.

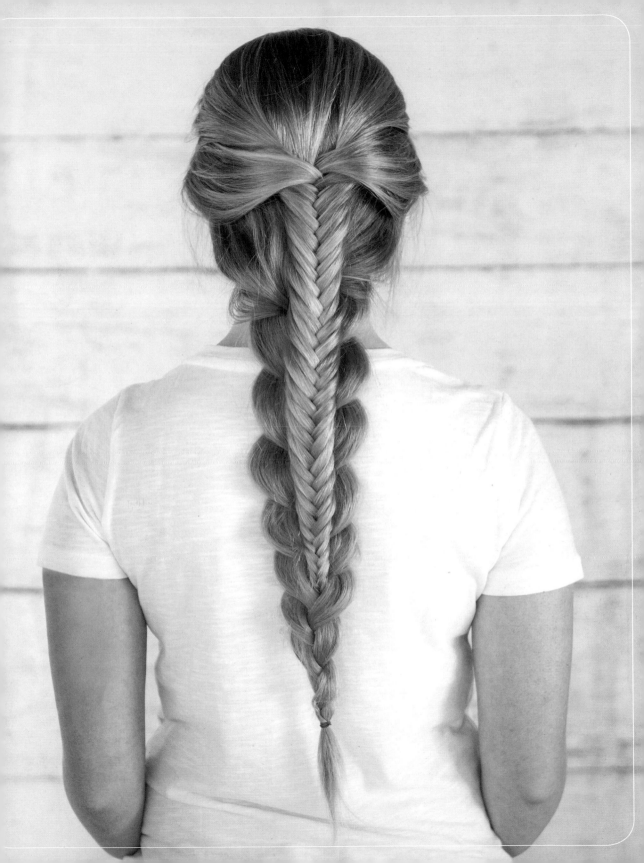

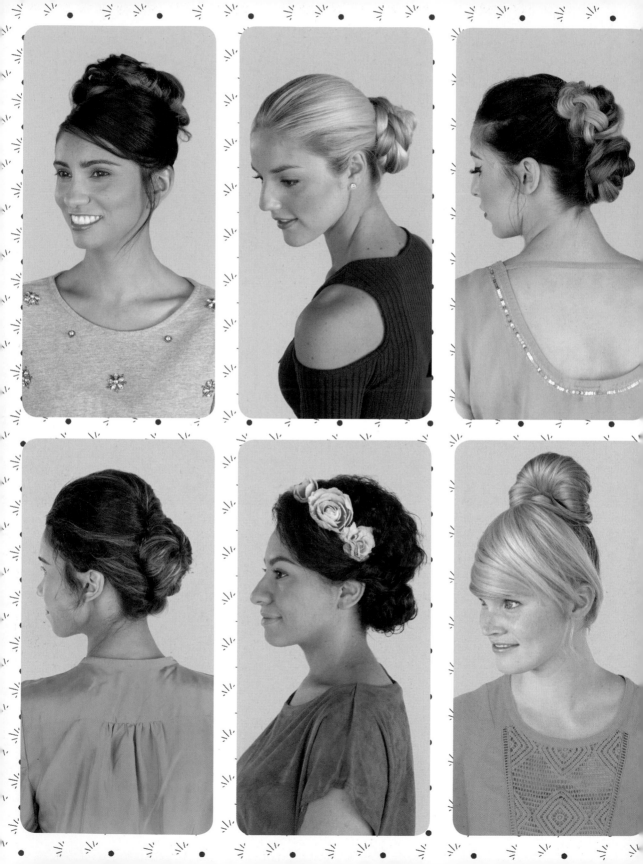

3

Buns

FAUX-FRINGE TOP KNOT

If you don't have a fringe and you're unsure about whether to get one, the faux-fringe top knot will give you the perfect trial run. This style will have you out the door in under five minutes, with a whole new do – and all the benefits of a fringe without the commitment! All you'll need is a comb and some hair bands, although you can make this fun and flirty by adding a jewelled headband.

1. Start by gathering your hair into a high ponytail. Secure it with a hair band.

2. Now create the basis for your faux fringe by folding the ponytail over so that its ends are pointing down towards your face.

3. Secure the loop formed by attaching another hair band at the base of the fold.

4. Now gently spread the looped hair out evenly, which will result in a fuller, more fanned-out bun.

5. Finally, comb the hair that was left out of the loop forwards to create your faux fringe.

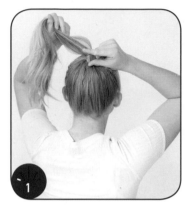

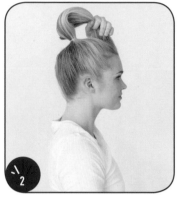

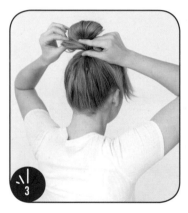

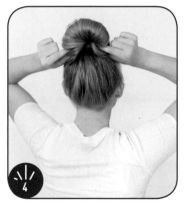

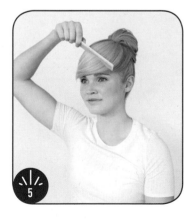

tip

If your hair is really straight after creating the faux fringe, try using straighteners to create a more natural bend.

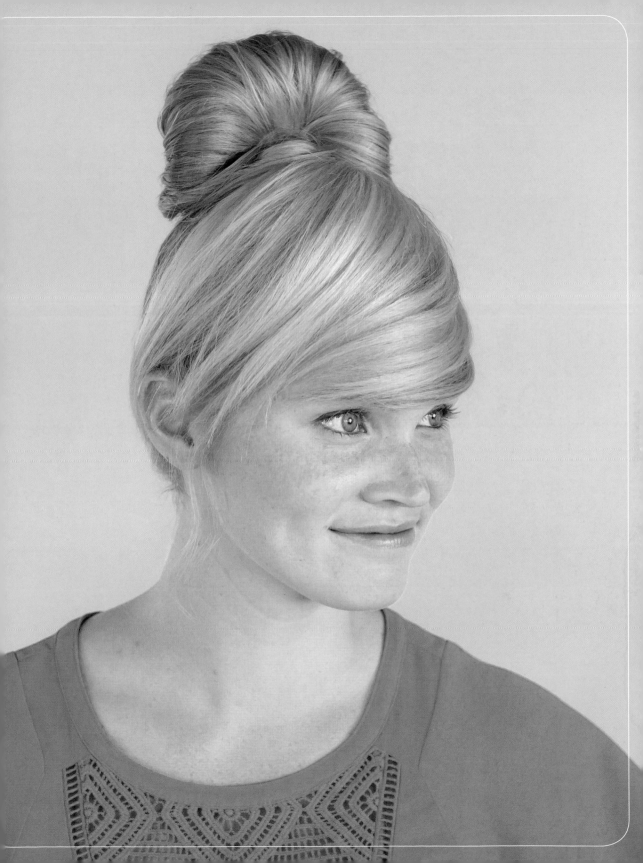

TWIST-AND-TUCK BUN

This flirty summer look comes together in no time at all. We've used a floral headband, but you can easily dress this look down with a simpler design. Just make sure your band extends all the way round your head. (This one has ties at the back.) For an even more effortless look, leave some strands hanging loose and curl them. Best of all? A headband and some pins are all you'll need!

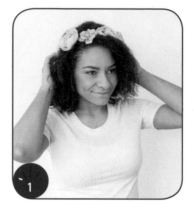

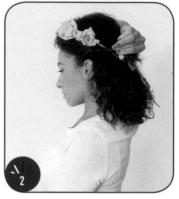

1. Pick out your favourite headband and secure it on your head. Make sure the headband is on top of your hair, not underneath it.

2. Now take two small strands (5–8cm/2–3in) from just above each ear and twist them away from your face.

3. Begin to tuck the ends into your headband. The closer you tuck them into the band, the tighter the finished bun will be.

4. Continue taking small sections and tucking them into your headband. Pull on the sections if you want to make the tucks look a bit fuller.

5. When all your hair has been incorporated, secure the twists with a few hair grips. If you have more layers, you may need a few extra hair grips!

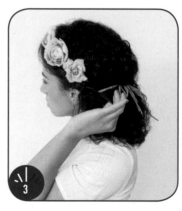

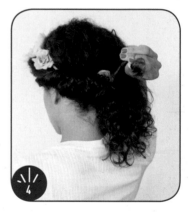

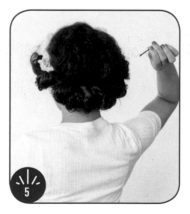

tip

Make sure to pick out a headband that fits you well. This will make it easier for the headband to hold your hair securely in place.

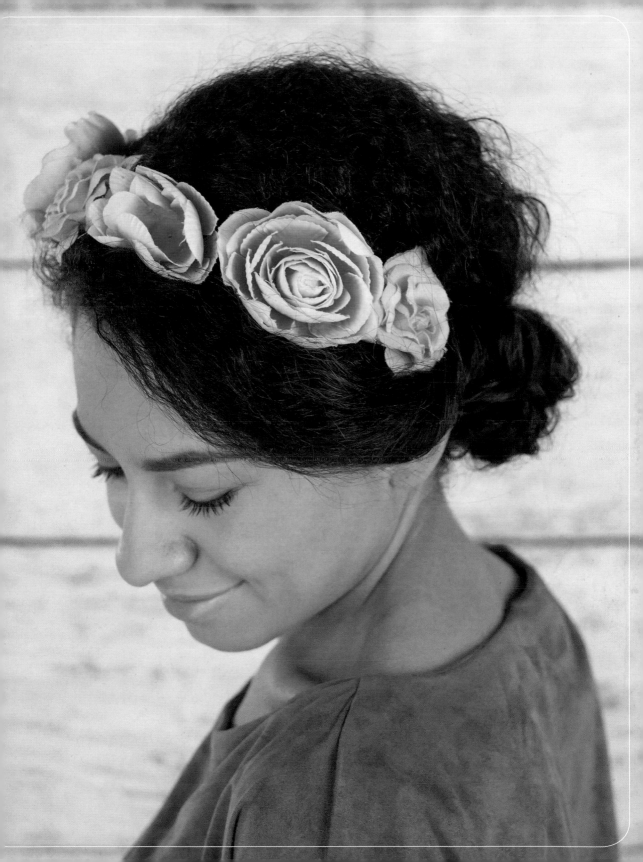

DOUBLE-PLAITED BUN

The double-plaited bun is a sexy and bold hairstyle. Ideal for long hair, this show-stopping style only takes a few minutes to create. To make it even more edgy, backcomb the roots of your hair for added volume. Leave some strands of hair down for a more casual vibe, or curl the loose strands for a special occasion. You will need four hair bands, a few hair grips and some hairspray.

1. Divide your hair in half horizontally, from ear to ear.

2. Comb the bottom section of hair into a low ponytail. Then just above this, comb the second section into a mid-ponytail.

3. Create a simple three-strand plait with the bottom ponytail and secure the ends with a hair band. Do the same with the upper ponytail.

4. Now 'pancake' each plait to create a dishevelled, more textured look.

5. To finish, wrap the top plait around the hair band at the base of the plait. Pin it in place with hair grips. Repeat this process for the bottom plait, then give everything a light mist of hairspray.

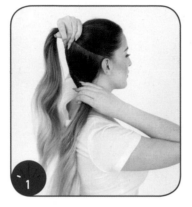

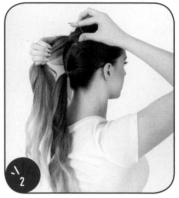

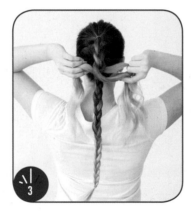

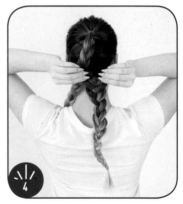

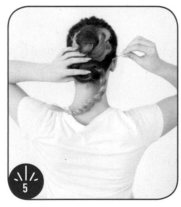

tip

To create a lighter feel, massage around the hairline with the palms of your hands after you have created your bun. This will give your hair a softer, more uneven texture.

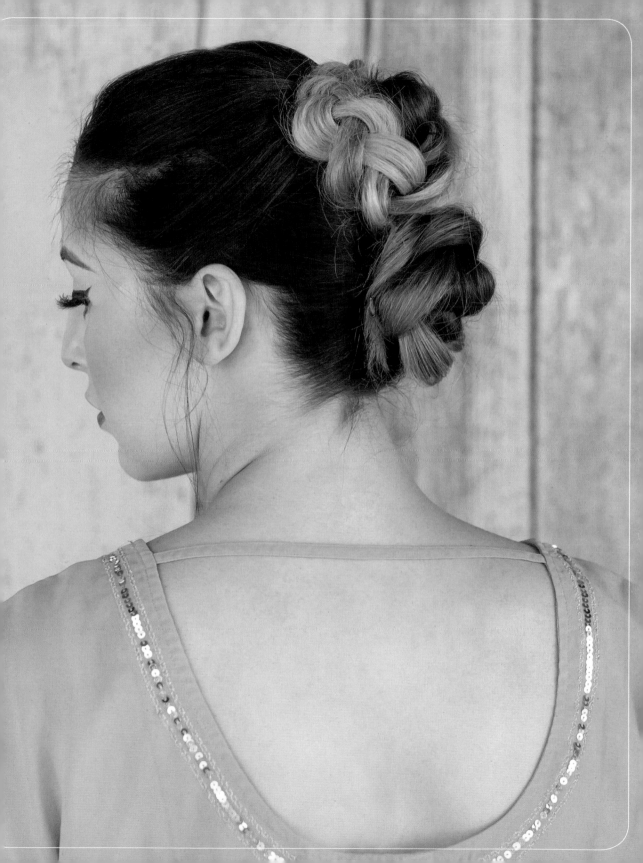

HALF-UP ROPE-PLAIT TOP KNOT

This top knot is perfect for those of you who struggle with keeping long hair out of your face. It is a great twist on the typical top knot, achieved with very little extra effort! The best thing about this look is that you can vary the plaits to suit your mood and personal style. And all you'll need are minimal tools – two hair bands, a hair clip, a few hair grips and a comb.

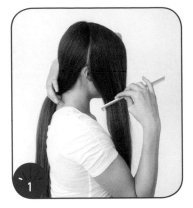

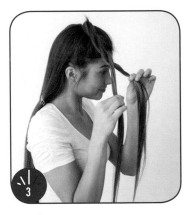

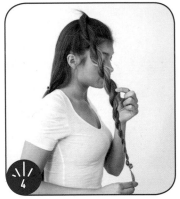

1. Separate your hair horizontally from ear to ear. Clip the lower section out of the way for now.

2. Comb the top section of hair towards the high-crown area and secure it in place with a hair band.

3. Divide this ponytail into two equal sections. Create a twist by following steps 3 and 4 on page 52, and secure the twist with a hair band when you've reached your desired length.

4. Holding on to the end of your rope plait, pinch and pull at random sections of it, tugging them in the direction of the base of the ponytail, to create a thicker appearance.

5. Now release your lower section of hair, then take your thickened rope plait, wrap it around the hair band, then secure it with hair grips.

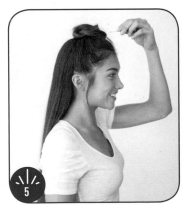

tip

Depending on how thick your hair is, you can include more or less hair in your ponytail to create a fatter or thinner top knot.

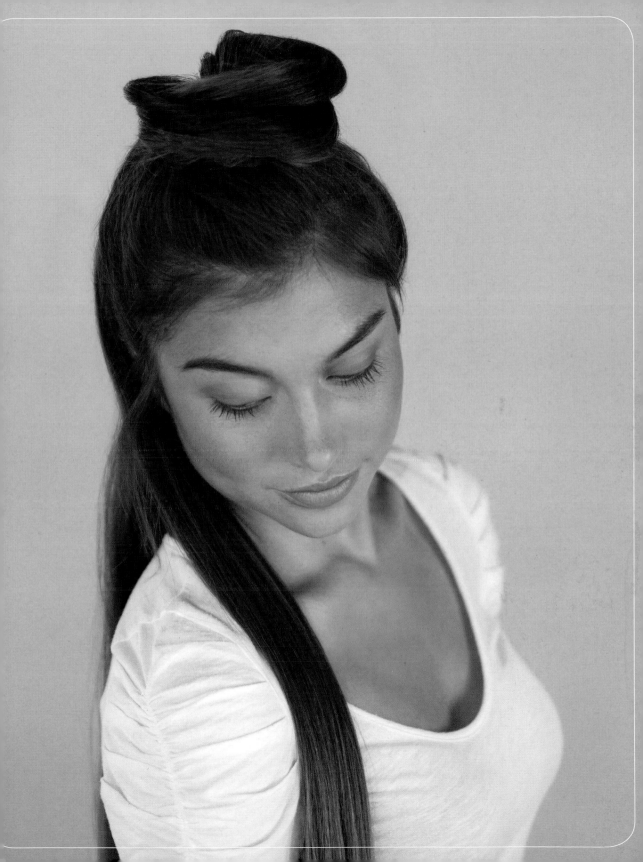

PLAITED BUN

You can never go wrong with this effortless, classic style. Wear it to mask your second-day hair, or create a clean and formal look right after a fresh wash. Either way, these five steps will have your hair looking amazing in no time! Make sure you have a comb, a couple of hair bands and a bunch of hair grips on hand before you start.

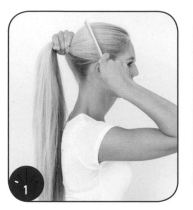
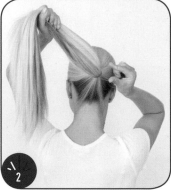

1. Comb through your hair thoroughly and then gather it all at the nape of your neck to create a low ponytail.

2. Secure the pony with a hair band, making sure the rest of your hair remains smooth.

3. Divide the ponytail into three equal sections and create a simple three-strand plait, securing it at the end with another hair band.

4. Now 'pancake' the plait a bit to create more fullness.

5. Finish by wrapping the plait around the base of the ponytail to create your plaited bun. Pin it in place in a circular pattern using as many hair grips as you need to hold it securely.

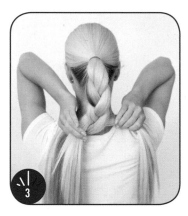
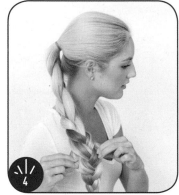

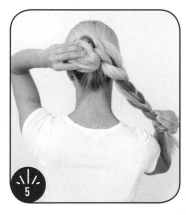

tip

If you're creating this look for a special occasion, try curling your hair before styling to give it a bit of extra interest and flair.

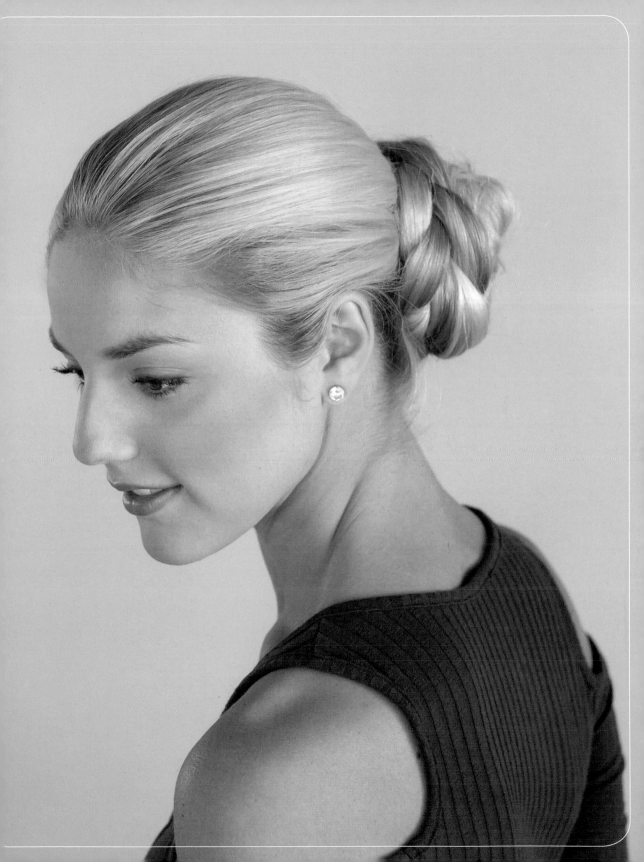

BOUFFANT INTO BACK BUN

This is another classic look that can be achieved in mere minutes and will keep your hair up and out of your face all day! Backcombing your roots a little and then adding a few twists results in a demure style that is perfect for work or a stylish brunch. As always, tools are very simple – you will only need a comb, hair clips and a small handful of hair grips.

1. Start by separating out a large section of hair on top of your head, from the forehead back to your high crown.

2. Keep the lower section out of the way for now with a clip or two. Meanwhile, working on your upper section, take 2.5cm (1in) portions and begin backcombing the roots aggressively. Continue backcombing until you've achieved your desired volume.

3. Now brush this whole section of hair out with your fingers while also pulling the hair back and forming a twist. Secure it in place with hair grips.

4. Release the lower section of hair, twist it from the roots to the ends, then create a low bun. Secure this with grips.

5. To add a bit more fullness, hold on to your bun and lightly pull on the bouffant.

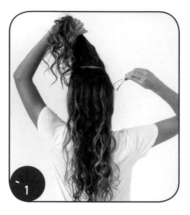

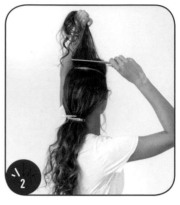

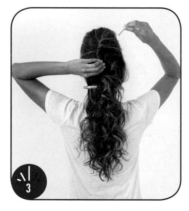

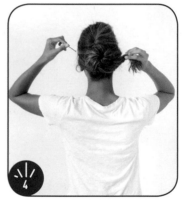

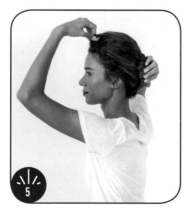

tip

Backcombing can make your hair prone to flyaways, so use a shine spray if this is a problem for your hair.

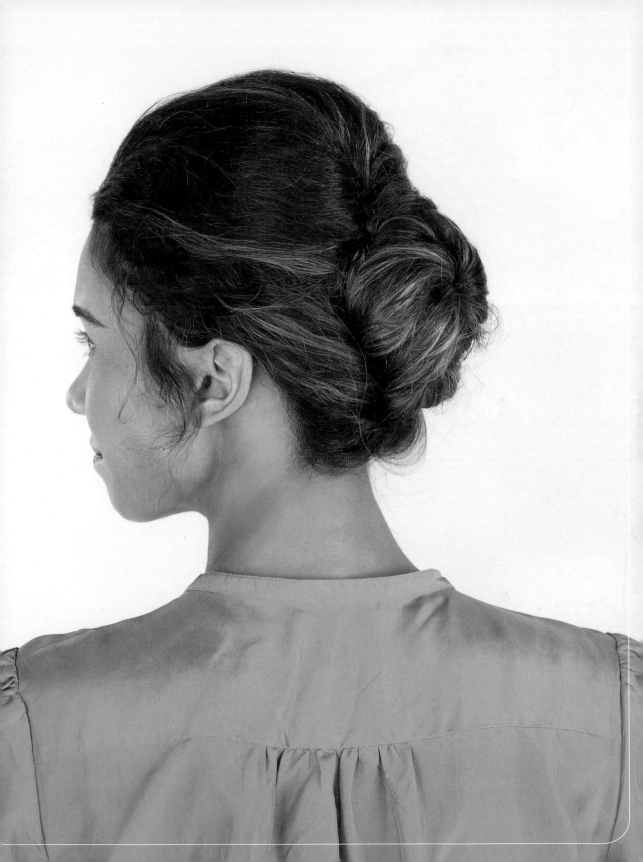

TWISTED TOP KNOT

Stay cute and flirty all day long with the twisted top knot! Whether you are having a lazy day or are a girl on the go, this is the perfect way to get your hair out of your face with minimal effort. If you want to make this look more formal, try it half-up half-down, and then curl the hair that hangs free. A hair band, a few hair grips and a comb are all you'll need to hand.

1. Comb your hair back tightly and up into your high-crown area.

2. Secure your hair into a high ponytail using a hair band.

3. Now pull this ponytail directly up and, holding it taut, twist it from the roots to the ends.

4. Give your twist some extra bulk and texture by grabbing bits of hair from the twist and pulling them down towards the base of the ponytail.

5. Finish off the look by creating a bun. Take the twisted ponytail and wrap it around the hair band, and then secure it in place with a handful of hair grips.

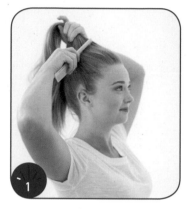

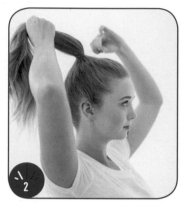

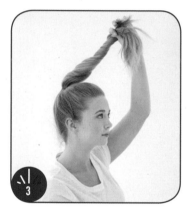

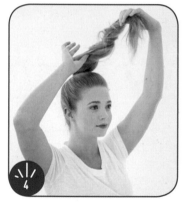

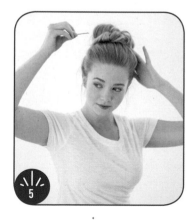

tip

If your hair lacks texture, 'grit' it up by using a texturising spray first. This will give your bun a more consistent and longer-lasting fullness.

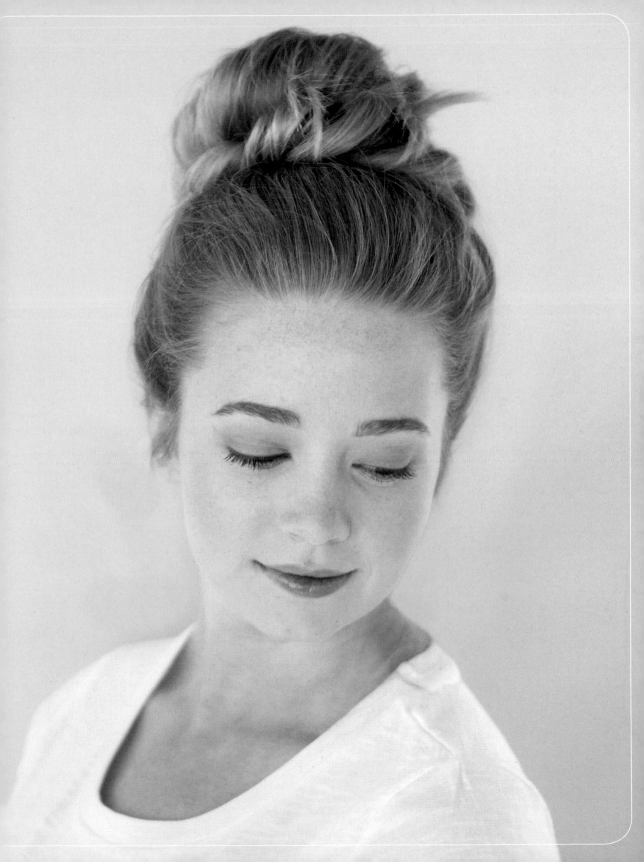

FORMAL TOP BUN

Once you've mastered this classic, you'll have a go-to look for dates, weddings and everything in between! As glamorous as it looks, it can be created with just a few simple moves. Forming the curls may take a while to begin with, but you will soon be whipping them up in no time at all. You will need a comb, curling tongs, some hair bands, hair grips and hairspray.

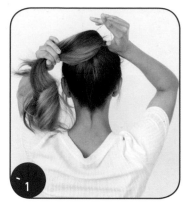

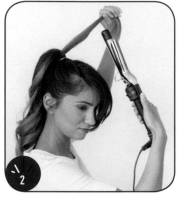

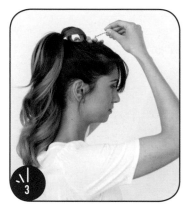

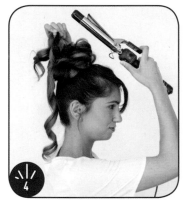

1. Gather your hair up into a high-crown ponytail and secure it with a hair band.

2. Take a portion of hair from the ponytail and curl it from the roots to the ends, leaving it on the curling tongs for a few seconds. If you have plenty of time and want a more intricate look, select a 2.5–5cm (1–2in) section. Curl larger section if you only have five minutes.

3. Carefully release the curl from the curling tongs, maintaining its curl, and pin it in place. Curls should be arranged to form a bun.

4. Continue this technique, securing curled sections around your hair band until all your hair has been curled. (Or save time if you like by opting to leave some strands hanging loose outside the bun.)

5. Make sure everything is held firmly with grips, then finish with a spritz of hairspray.

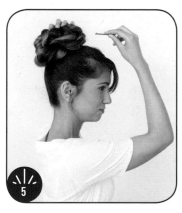

tip

This is a great style whether you have a fringe or not! If you do, you can either pin it back, or curl it and leave it down.

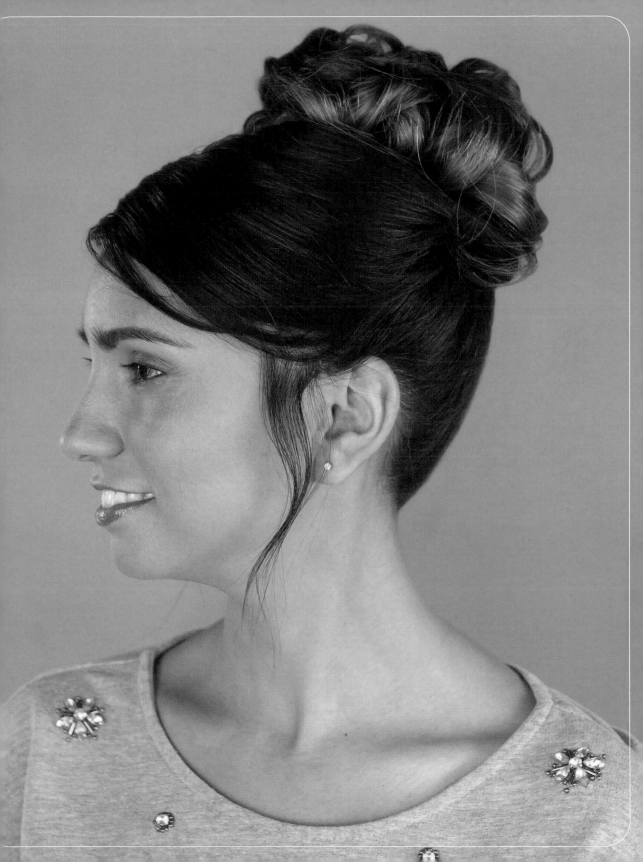

TRIPLE MESSY BUN

The triple messy bun will give you a super-cool twist on your everyday messy bun. This casual look is done in minutes but it can be worn all day long – it's meant to be messy, so there is no need to worry about trying to keep it perfectly in place throughout the day. As usual, simple tools are all you'll need: hair bands, hair grips and a comb.

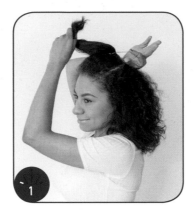

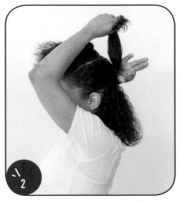

1. Take a small horseshoe-shaped section from the top of your head, with the parting reaching back to the crown area. Create a small ponytail by securing the hair with a hair band.

2. Clip away your first ponytail for now, then take a horizontal section of hair from ear to ear to create a second ponytail. The third ponytail can then be created with the hair remaining below this.

3. Now take the first ponytail and tightly twist it from the base to the ends. Create a top knot by wrapping the twist around the base of the hair band.

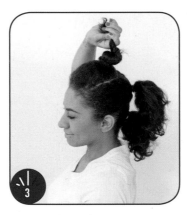

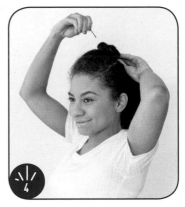

4. Secure the first bun in place with hair grips, then create top knots in the same way with the remaining two ponytails.

5. For the final touch, pinch and pull each bun out gently to create a messier, fuller look.

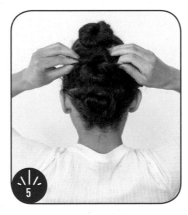

tip

If you have straight hair that lacks fullness and texture, just add some curls before starting.

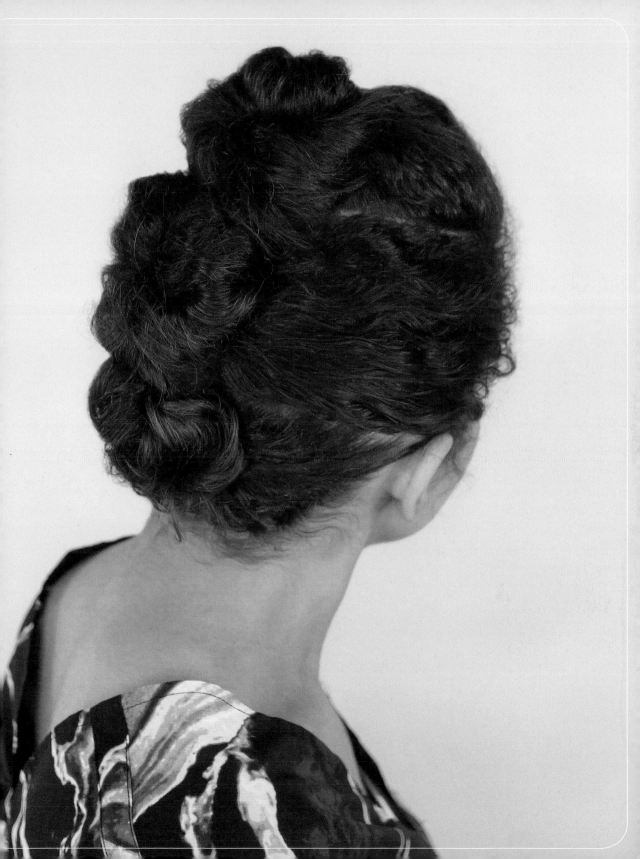

KNOTTED BACK BUN

The knotted back bun is a trendy way to make a bun. It's fun, flirty and totally different. Wear this to a concert or just out and about – like so many styles in this book, it's a look that is incredibly versatile. And, of course, it can be created in no time at all. Grab hair bands, a comb and a few hair grips and give it a go!

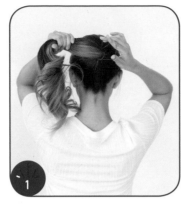
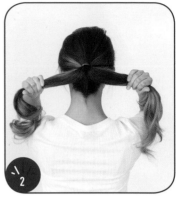

1. Gather your hair at the back of your head and create a ponytail. Secure it firmly with a hair band.

2. Comb out the ponytail and then divide the hair into two equal sections.

3. Now take these two sections of hair and tie them into a knot.

4. Continue tying the two sections of hair into knots until you reach the ends, then secure the knotted plait that you've created with a hair band.

5. Finally, wrap the knotted plait around the base of the ponytail to create a bun, and use hair grips to hold it firmly in place.

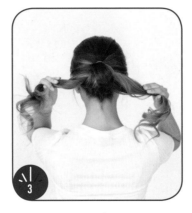
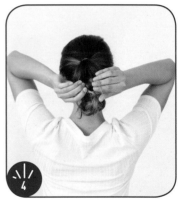
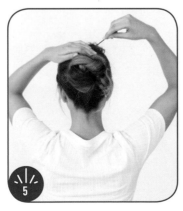

tip

If you fancy more of an effortless style, take the knotted plait and gently rub it between the palms of your hands before you create the bun. This will give you a more bohemian look.

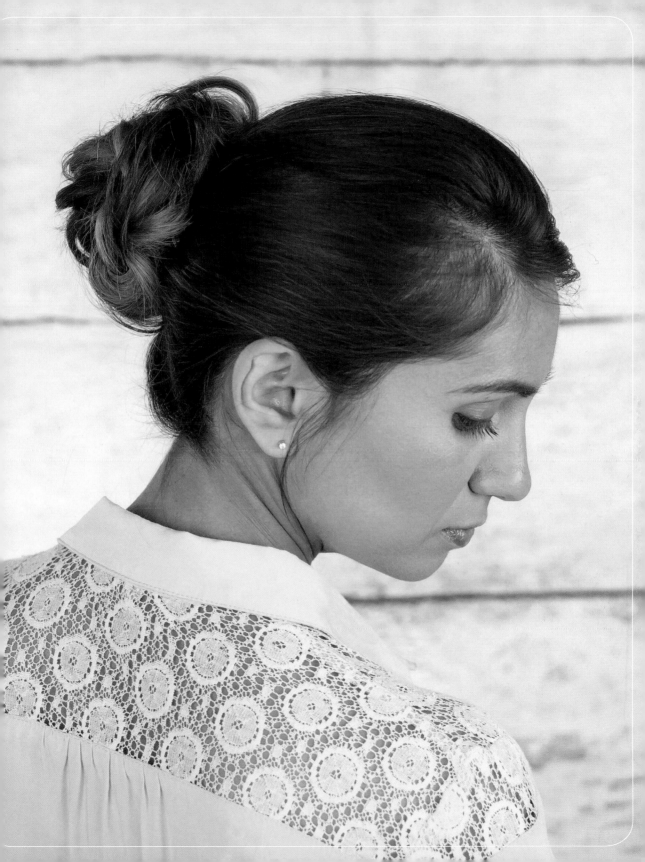

LOW SNAKE-COIL BUN

This chic style looks good on everyone and yet it requires hardly any effort at all. In fact, lots of women coil their hair up into a snake-coil bun without even realising that's what they're doing! The only items that you'll need are some hair bands, a comb, a few hair grips and some hairspray, but feel free to spice this look up with some hair accessories if the mood calls for it.

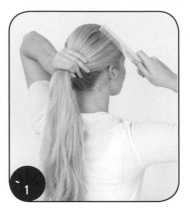

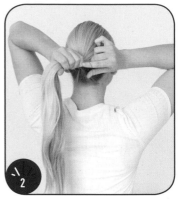

1. Comb your hair back evenly to the nape of your neck.

2. Secure this low ponytail with a hair band.

3. Now twist the ponytail from the base to the tip as tightly as possible in order to create your snake coil.

4. Let the twist naturally coil around your hair band to create a bun and then use hair grips to hold it in place. Use three to four grips distributed evenly around the bun for maximum support.

5. Finish off by applying a bit of hairspray and then very gently comb through to get rid of any flyaways and create a sleeker look at your roots.

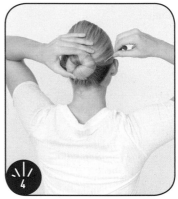

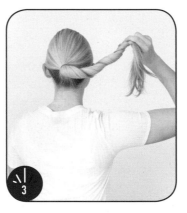

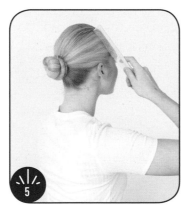

tip

If your hair is naturally curly or wavy, you can get a sleeker finish by round-brushing or straightening your hair before you begin.

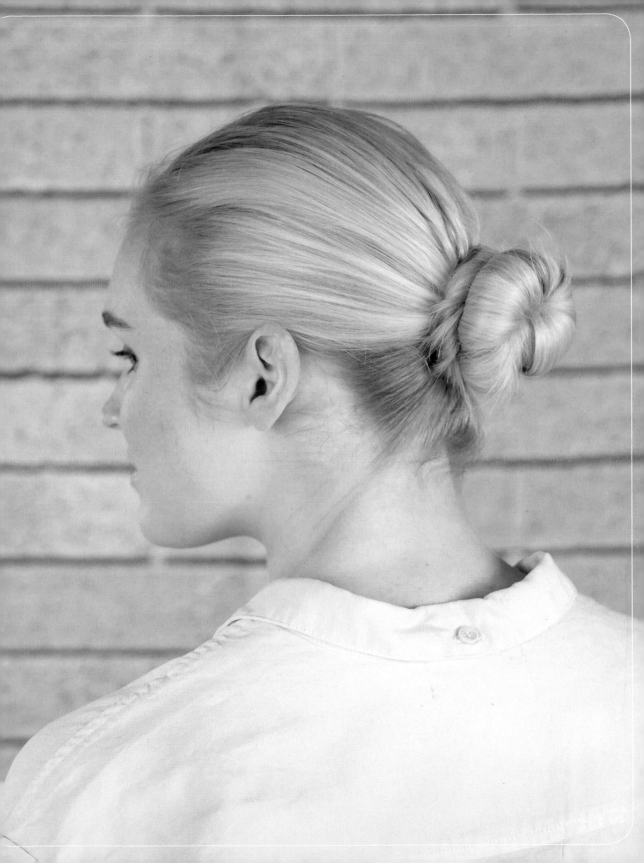

LOW BUN WITH PLAITED HEADBAND

The low bun with plaited headband is a boho-chic way to deal with that second-day hair, and one that, with practice, only takes a few minutes. Wear it casually or for a formal event – everyone will love how it looks, and you'll love how little time it takes to create! Simply grab a few hair bands, a comb and a handful of hair grips and you'll be ready to begin.

1. Take a 5–8cm (2–3in) section of hair from behind one ear.

2. Now use this section to create a simple plait and secure the end with a hair band. Repeat steps 1 and 2 on the other side of your head.

3. Gather the rest of your hair to the nape of your neck and use a hair band to form a ponytail.

4. Twist the ponytail you have just created to form a bun (see pages 78–79), and then secure it firmly in place using a few hair grips.

5. The last step is to bring the right and left plaits over your head to create the plaited headband. Tuck the ends of each plait into your hair to conceal them, and secure them in place with grips.

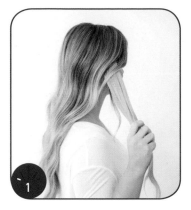

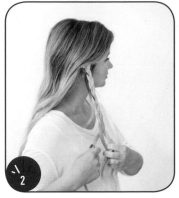

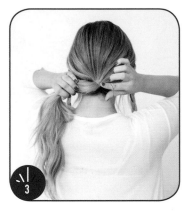

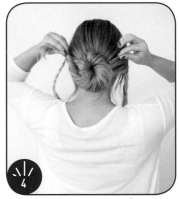

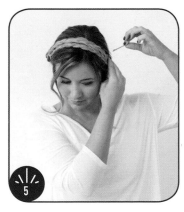

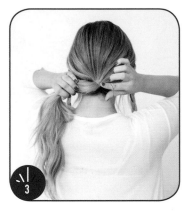

tip

Get creative with your plaits! See if you can find ways of making this style your own by mixing it up a bit and using different types of plait.

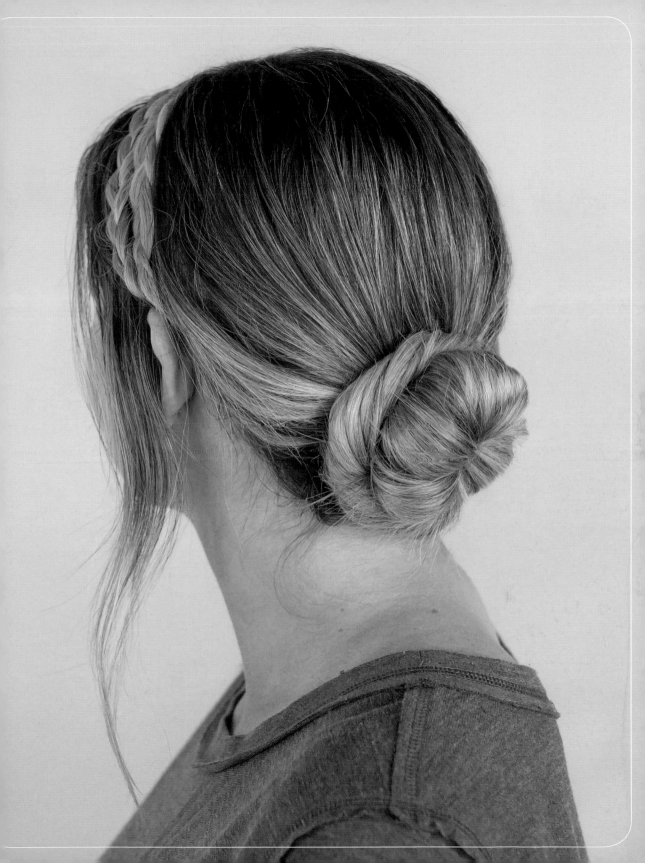

PLAIT-WRAPPED TOP KNOT

The plait-wrapped top knot is a real classic. Not only is this style simple to create, it is also easy to morph from casual to special occasion, which is what makes it such a lasting favourite. This quick and efficient 'do can be rocked from the beach to the dance floor in just a few quick moves! Grab a comb, a couple of hair bands, a hair clip and a few hair grips, and let's get started.

1. Gather all of your hair into the high-crown area and secure it in place with a hair band.

2. Depending on how thick your hair is, take a 2.5–5cm (1–2in) section of hair from the ponytail you've just created and clip it out of the way for now.

3. Twist the rest of the ponytail from roots to ends and wrap it around the hair band to create a top knot (see pages 78-79).

4. Secure the top knot in place with hair grips.

5. Now take the sectioned-off hair and create a simple three-strand plait, securing the end with a hair band. Then wrap the plait around the base of your top knot and secure it with some more grips.

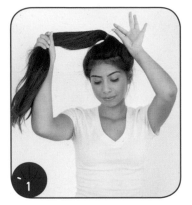

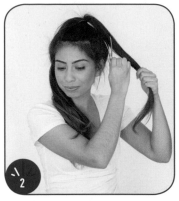

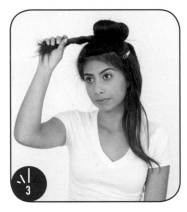

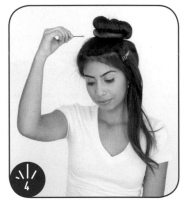

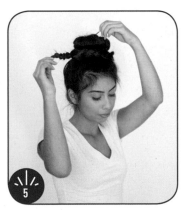

tip

If you don't have hair long enough to wrap around your top knot, use a hair extension and plait it to create the plait instead.

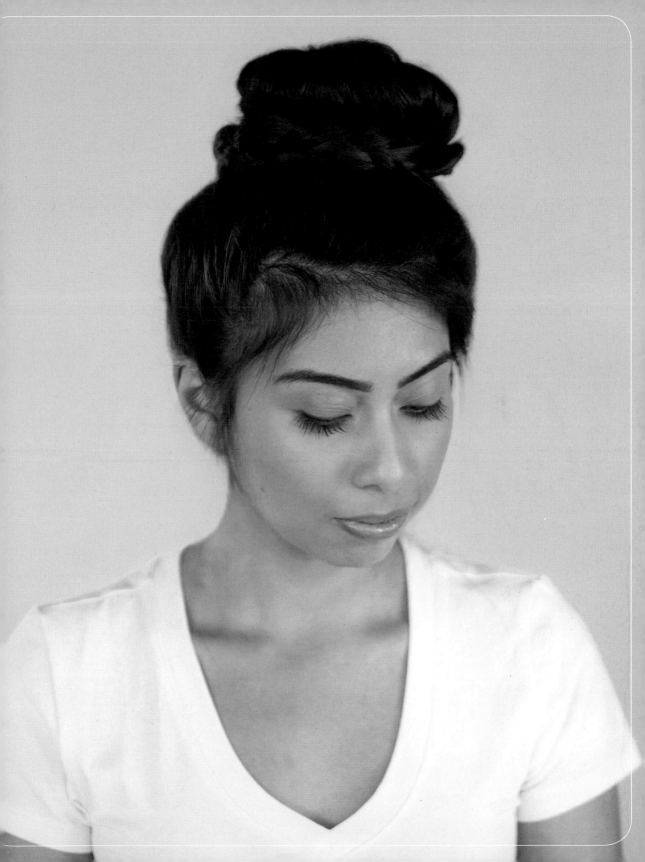

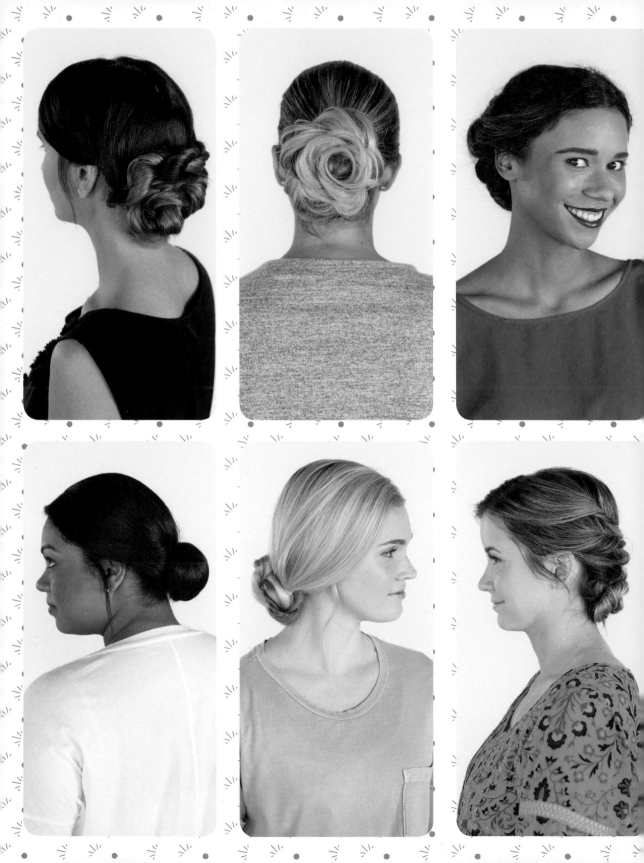

4

Party Updos

ROPE-PLAIT UPDO

The rope-plait updo is a wonderful style to master – with the aid of just a comb, some clips, hair bands and hair grips, a few simple twists will set you up for an amazing night out in just minutes! You can also downplay this look and create a more bohemian effect by pulling out the twists in the rope plait, or by leaving some strands out of the plait altogether.

1. Section out some hair at the back of your head from the crown to mid-ear, then clip the top sections out of the way.

2. Create a low ponytail, then begin your rope plait. Divide the pony into two equal sections. Twist the right section clockwise, then bring it up and over the left section (see page 52). Repeat this process until you have your desired length of plait.

3. Now wrap your rope plait around the elastic to create a bun and secure it with grips.

4. Release the clip on one side of your head and divide this section in half to create another rope plait. Secure it with a hair band, then repeat on the other side.

5. Drape one side plait over and around your bun and secure it in place with a grip, then do the same with the other side.

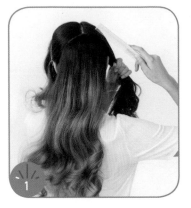

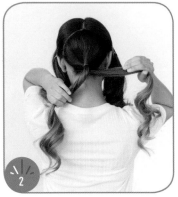

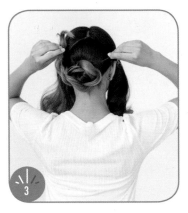

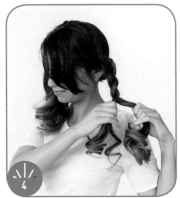

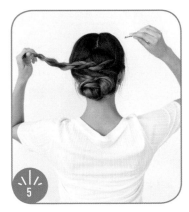

tip

When plaiting the sides, twist them away from your face and then intertwine the sections in the opposite direction to the one that you twisted them in.

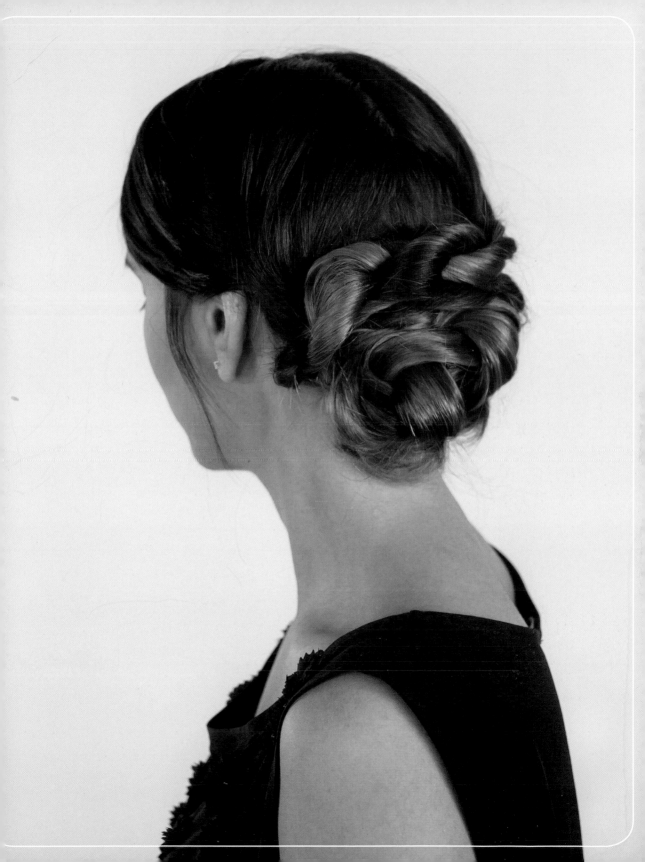

TOPSY-TAIL TUCK ROLL

The topsy-tail tuck roll is an elegant, discreet hairstyle that flatters everyone. It can be worn to a party or on a date –either way, you are bound to attract attention! This style works best on mid-length, medium to thick hair, but it suits all ages, and you can add some glamour with sparkly hair accessories. You'll need some hairspray, a comb, a hair band and some hair grips to create this.

1. Begin by pulling your hair back into a low ponytail and securing it with a hair band.

2. Separate the hair at the base of the ponytail, just above your hair band, to create a small hole. Lift the ponytail up and pass it through this hole, pulling it through completely. This action will cause the sides of your hair to roll inwards, creating a topsy-tail effect.

3. Now prepare a roll by wrapping the pony around the index and middle fingers of one hand until you have a shape you are happy with.

4. Hold the roll firmly in place with one hand while you use your free hand to secure it with plenty of hair grips.

5. Finish by combing down any flyaways and using hairspray to keep everything in place.

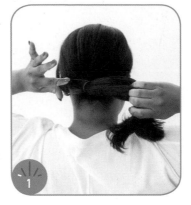

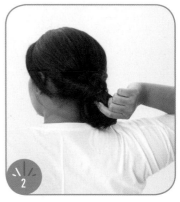

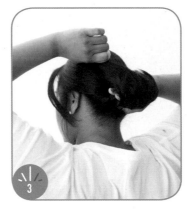

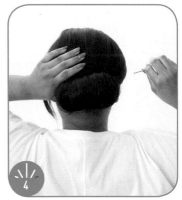

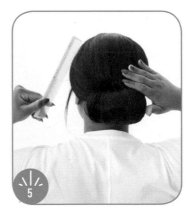

tip

If you have naturally straight hair, curl it prior to starting to help limit any flyaways.

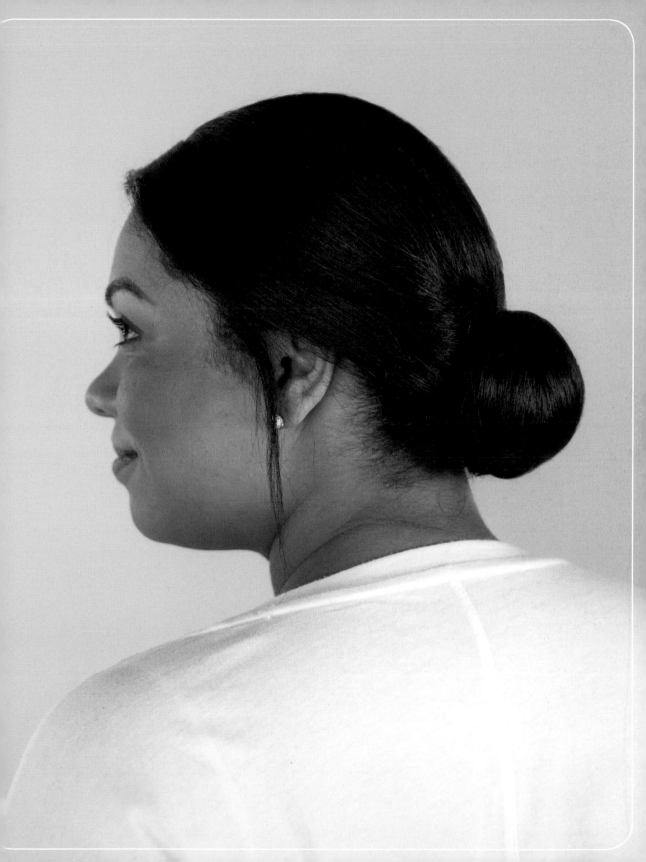

TWIST-AND-BACKCOMB LOW UPDO

The twist-and-backcomb low updo is the perfect look for a date – it takes under five minutes to do and can easily be dressed up by adding hair accessories. For example, try rocking this look during the day by going for a boho effect with some fake flowers or a floral headband. Otherwise, the basics you'll need for this look are a comb, two hair clips, some hair grips and a hair band.

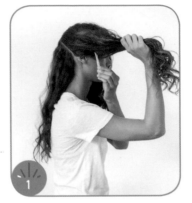
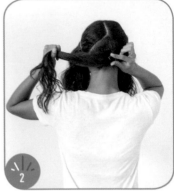

1. Begin by taking a section of hair running from your crown to mid-ear. Clip the upper sections to either side, out of the way for now.

2. Now create a low ponytail by gathering the hair at the nape of your neck and securing it with a hair band.

3. Next create your twist-and-backcomb effect by twisting your ponytail aggressively from the base and through to the ends.

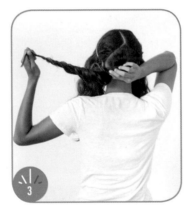
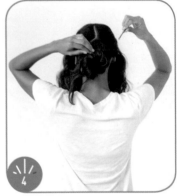

4. Wrap this twisted hair around the base of the hair band to create a bun, and secure it in place with some hair grips.

5. Now release your side sections from their clips. Twist both of these sections using the same technique as before, and then drape the pieces over the bun. Secure them in place with a few more hair grips.

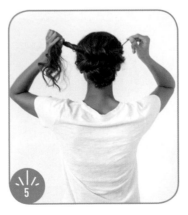

tip

If your hair is very thick, feel free to section out smaller pieces for your twists.

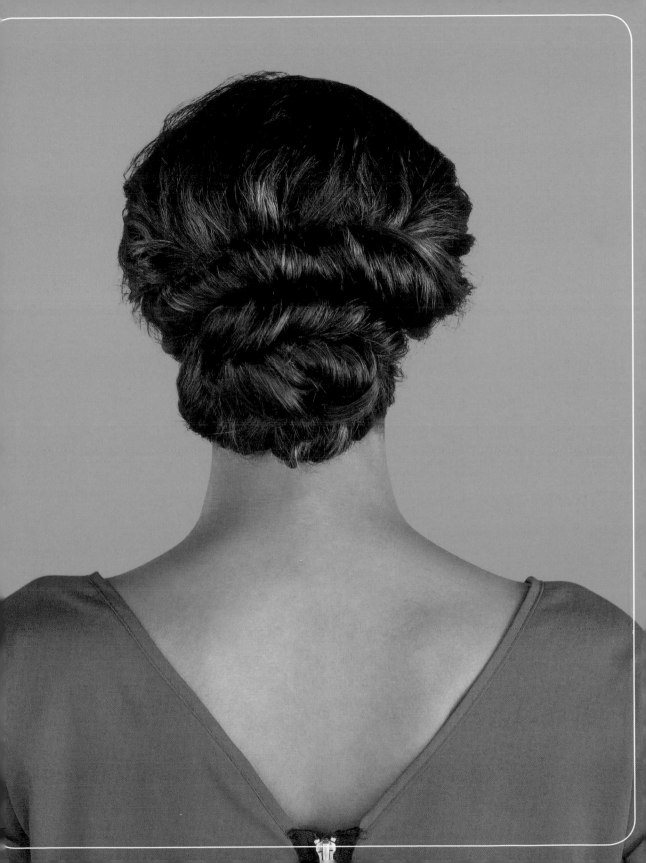

PULLED-OUT PLAITED UPDO

The sophistication and detail of this look make it striking enough to wear to important events, and you'll be amazed when you discover just how easy it is to create. You can also give it a more edgy look by backcombing your hair prior to styling, and by pulling hair out of the plait more vigorously. Make sure you have a comb, a few hair grips and a hair band to hand before you start.

1. Working from the temples back to the crown of the head, take a horseshoe-shaped section of hair.

2. Divide this into three equal strands. Start creating a Dutch plait by taking the right strand under and into the middle, then take the left strand under and into the middle.

3. Now incorporate a 2.5cm (1in) section of hair into the right strand before bringing it under and into the middle. Repeat on the left side. Continue in this way until all your hair is incorporated, then continue the plait to the ends. Secure it with a hair band.

4. Stretch the plait out vigorously to create volume and texture.

5. Finish by creating your bun. Flip the plait under and then secure it with grips, arranging it in a rounded shape.

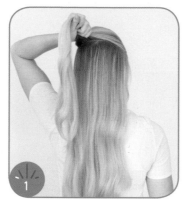

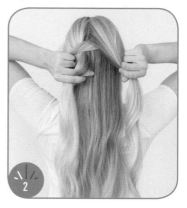

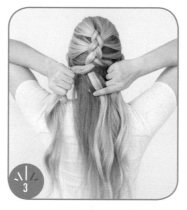

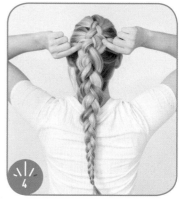

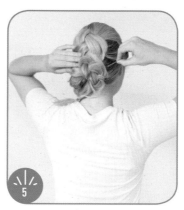

tip

If you decide to create a looser plait by pulling the strands out further, make sure you anchor the bun well with hair grips for longer-lasting fullness.

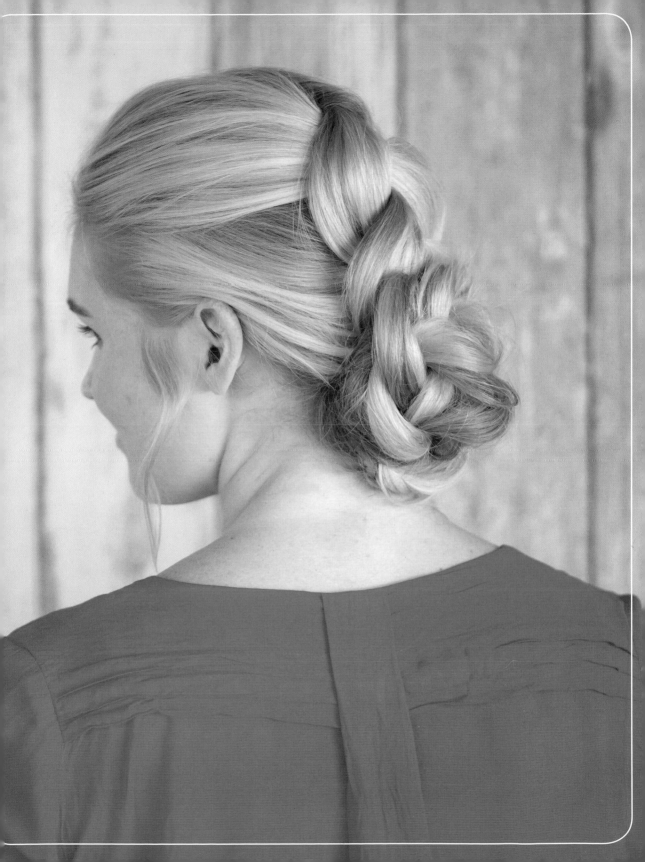

LOW FLOWER UPDO

If you know how to create a simple three-strand plait then you will be able to create the low flower updo. This is yet another hairstyle that looks more complicated than it is – and who doesn't love that? If your hair is dirty and you're in a pinch, do this look to the side and then throw on a hat or a headband. Grab a comb, a couple of hair bands and some hair grips and let's work through the steps!

1. Begin by combing your hair towards the back of your head and secure it with a hair band.

2. Now divide the ponytail you've just created into three strands to create a simple plait.

3. When you reach the end of the plait, secure it with another hair band. Then, holding on to the plait from one side, pull and stretch out the opposing side to create volume. Do this down the length of the plait.

4. Take the side of the plait that hasn't been stretched out and wrap it tightly around the base of your pony. The stretched-out half of the plait should be sitting around the outside of the bun, creating your 'flower'.

5. Secure your plait in place using hair grips, maintaining a circular shape all the way around for the most realistic flower effect.

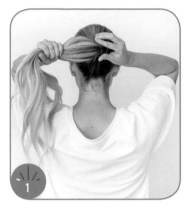

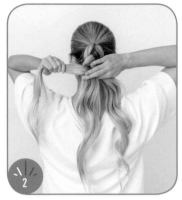

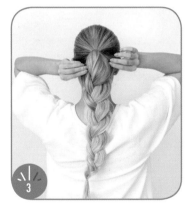

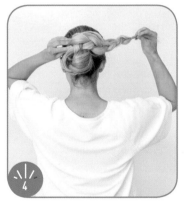

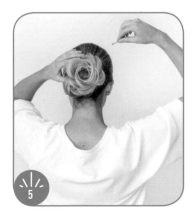

tip

If there are any straight ends of hair left out of the hair band once you've created your bun, try curling them so that they bend naturally around the flower.

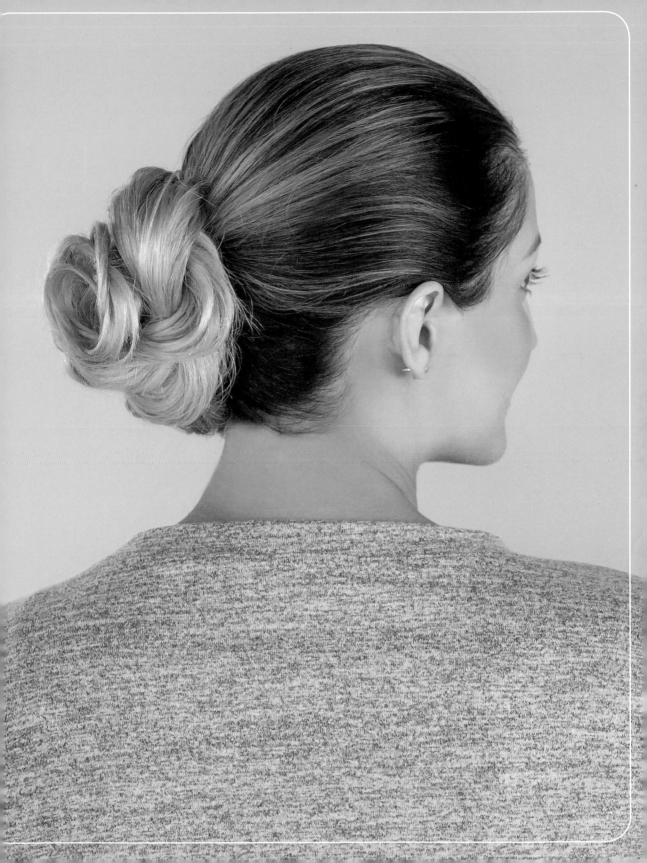

STACKED-TWISTS UPDO

If you're heading out and you're facing a time crunch, then look no further than the stacked-twists updo! Make this look formal or casual by starting out with either clean or textured hair. This look involves nothing more than a few easy twists, and you can really make it your own by embellishing it with accessories. Otherwise all you need is a comb and a few hair grips.

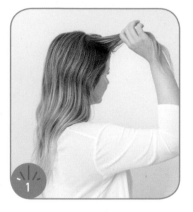

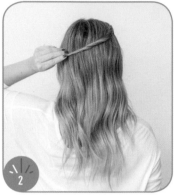

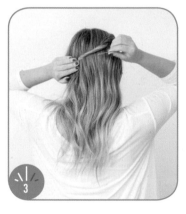

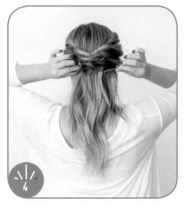

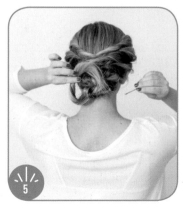

1. Part your hair on the desired side, then separate a horizontal section on one side (2.5–5cm/1–2in), working back from your hairline.

2. Twist this section of hair away from your face while directing it behind and towards the other side of your head.

3. Secure the twist with a grip.

4. Now take an equal-sized section from the other side of your head and repeat steps 2 and 3. Continue working your horizontal sections from right to left in the same way. Keep going until you have incorporated all the hair on both sides and have just a few strands remaining at the nape.

5. Take the very ends of the leftover strands, twist them and then pin them into the rest of the updo.

tip

This look is easily transformed into a half-up half-down style. Simply leave the remaining hair down after your desired number of twists. The result will be something like step 4.

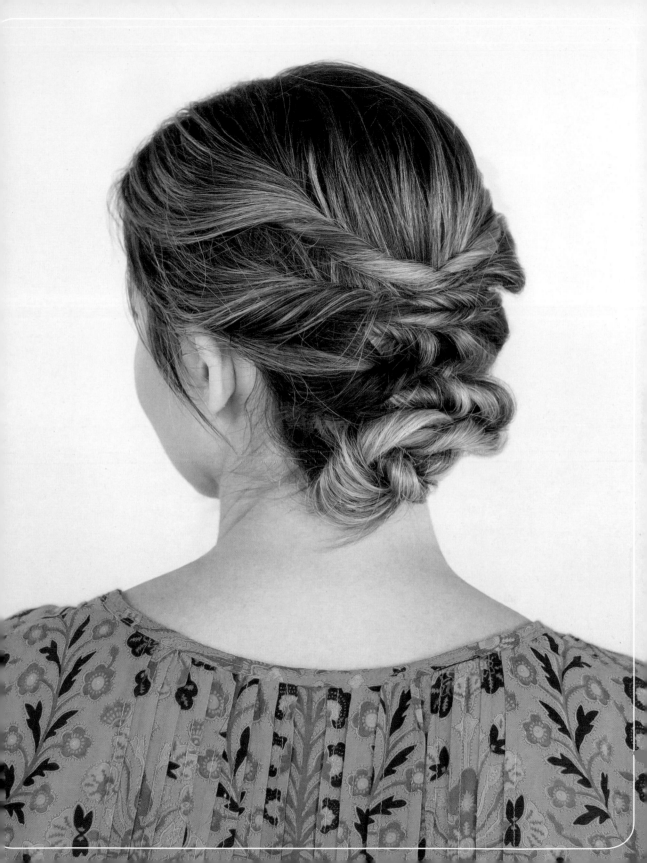

SIDE-KNOT UPDO

Heading out with just five minutes to spare? Not a problem – requiring just a comb, a hair band and a few hair grips, the side-knot updo gives you a quick and handy way to jazz up a traditional side plait. The knotted effect adds an interesting texture with no extra effort. If you want a more formal look, simply curl your hair, do the knot to the back and spritz on some shine spray.

1. Comb your hair to the desired side and then divide it into two equal sections.

2. Cross one section over the other, then pull it under and through the gap between them to create a simple knot.

3. Continue with this knotting technique until you've reached your desired length. When you're finished, secure the end of the plait with a hair band.

4. Now take the end of your knotted plait. Loop it around and then tuck it neatly inside the initial division of hair you made in step 1.

5. Finish by securing the loop in place with hair grips.

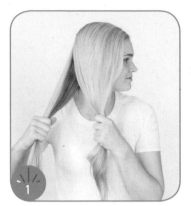

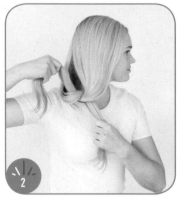

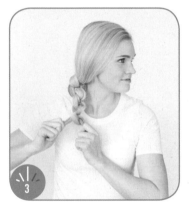

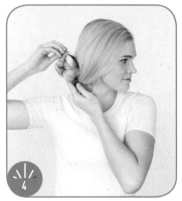

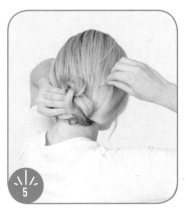

tip

If you want more volume in your updo, backcomb the roots of your hair prior to starting.

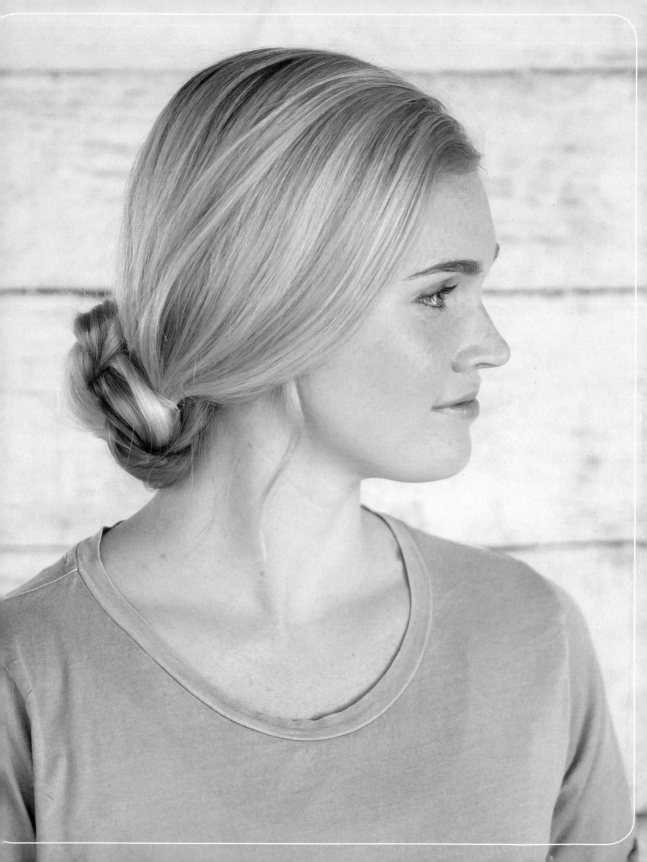

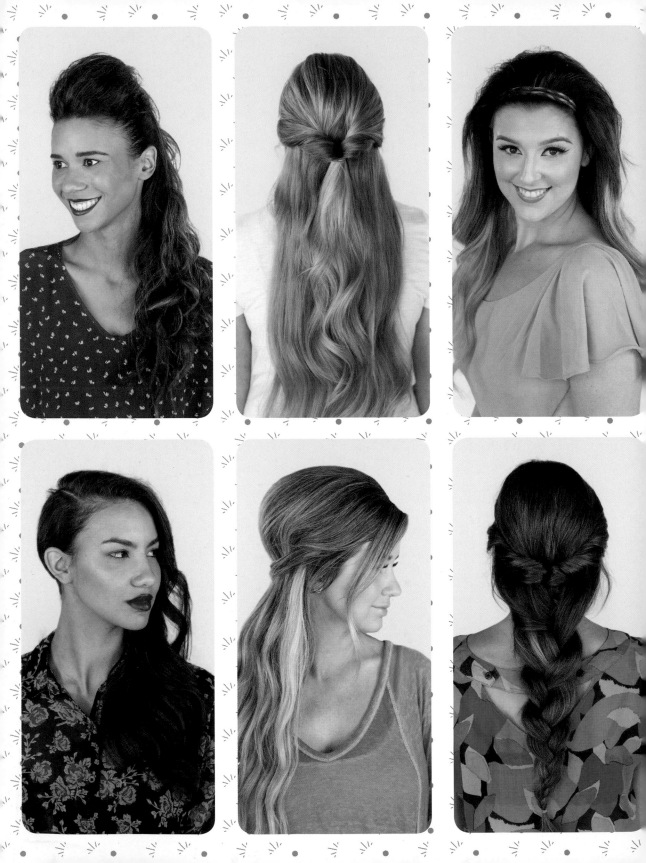

5

Down Styles

HALF-DOWN TWISTED TOPSY-TAIL

The half-down twisted topsy-tail is a quick style for a chic girl on the go. Wear the version shown here for errands, or curl it before heading out on that hot date – either way, this style will leave you looking and feeling fantastic! You can even plait the topsy-tail if you want to take things a step further. Best of all, a comb and a hair band are all you'll need to achieve this look.

1. Start by dividing your hair in half horizontally, parting it from ear to ear.

2. Now comb the top section into a ponytail and secure it with a hair band.

3. Divide this hair evenly in half at the base of the ponytail.

4. Take the ponytail and bring it up and down through the centre of the halved hair at the base. Pull the ponytail down and all the way through.

5. Finally, to exaggerate the twist and create a fuller look, carefully pull out small sections of the topsy-tail.

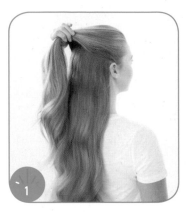

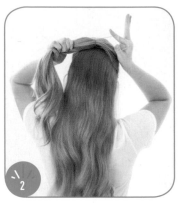

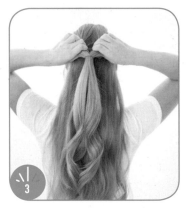

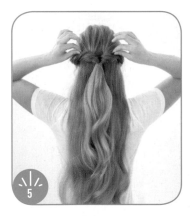

tip

If your hair is extremely fine and you want to rock this 'do, lightly curl your hair prior to styling. This will help add volume.

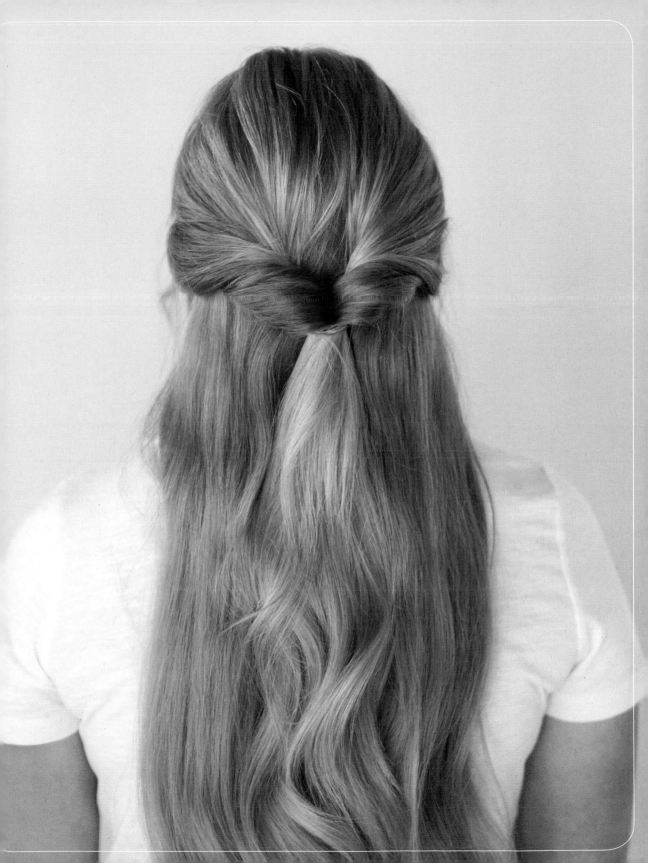

CURLY FRONT TWIST

This is a fun and fresh alternative to a French plait. Using a similar technique, you add strands of hair into your twist. However, using only two strands of hair instead of three makes it a much easier choice if you are unsure of how to plait, or only have limited time! You'll need a comb, some hair bands, a couple of hair grips, a hair clip and some curling tongs.

1. Part your hair to the desired side. Grab a small section at the front (5–8cm/2–3in) and create your first twist.

2. Take another small section of hair directly under the first one and incorporate it into the first twist. Twist it a couple of times. This will give the twist a better ridge at the hairline.

3. Continue incorporating new sections of hair into the twist until you reach your ear, then continue twisting the hair through to the ends. Clip this against your head for now.

4. Take a small section of hair from above where you would like to secure your twist and clip it out of the way. Pin the twist in place, then release the hair on top to conceal the grip.

5. Finish by using your curling tongs to add a quick curl or two if you want extra volume.

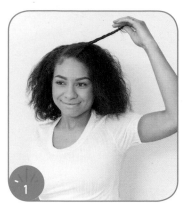

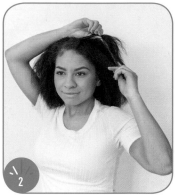

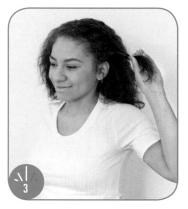

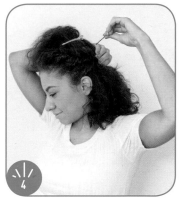

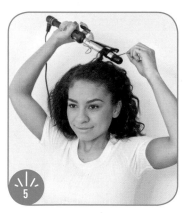

tip

If you have layers in your hair, or a lot of flyaways, try using a little pomade to keep the twist looking neat and fresh.

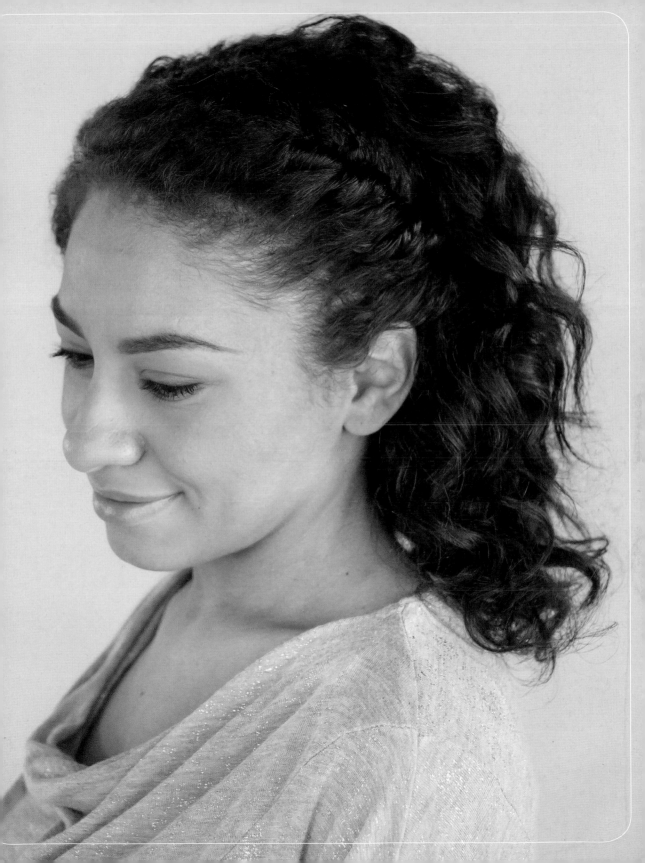

POMPADOUR

Although you will learn how to complete this 'do in hardly any time at all, the pompadour is one of the most diverse looks around. Wear it out on a date or with your best girls – with a little hair product and some backcombing, you'll be ready to rock your evening! Gather together a comb, a few hair clips, some hairspray and a hair band, and let's work through the process step by step.

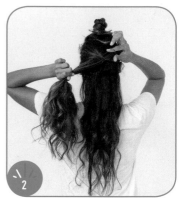

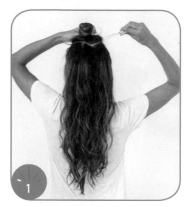

1. Begin by separating out a triangular section of hair at the top of your head and clip it out of the way for now.

2. Take a section from just above your right ear and do the same on your left, then gather these sections into the low-crown area and create a ponytail by securing them together with a hair band. Be sure to keep the sides smooth and tight.

3. Release the top triangular section and use your comb to backcomb your hair at the roots until you have created your desired volume.

4. Now lightly comb over the top of your hair to cover up the backcombing.

5. Finally, add some hairspray and comb through the sides to create a sleeker look.

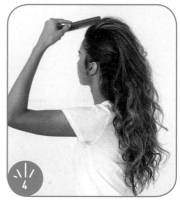

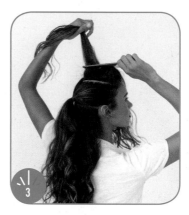

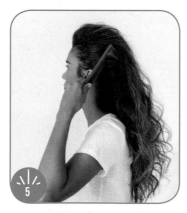

tip

If your hair is thick and heavy, simply use a few hair grips to help maintain the volume.

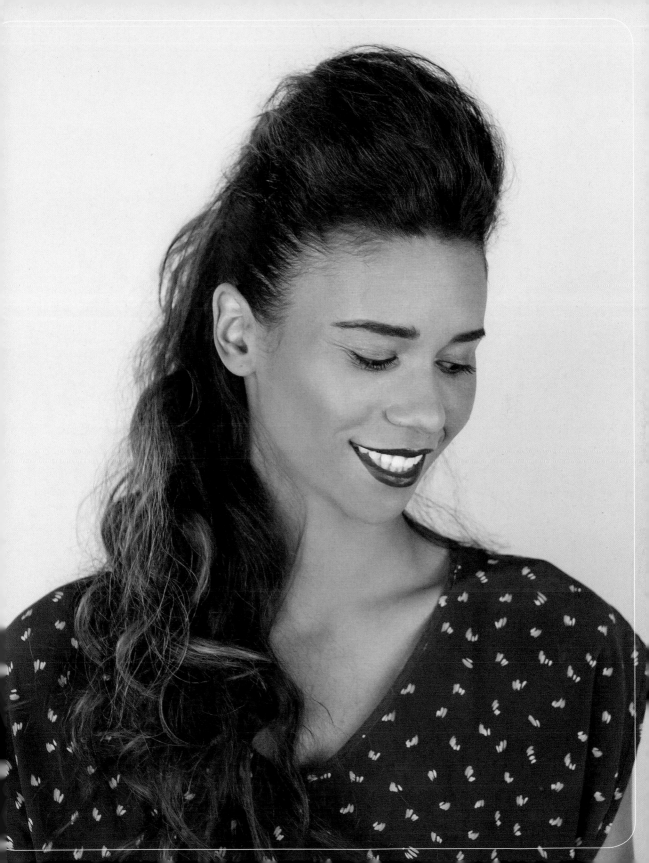

BOUFFANT WITH PLAITED HEADBAND

While there are many hairstyles that should remain in the 1970s, this inspired look is certainly not one of them. The plaits add a flirty modern twist, and the volume at the crown of your head can be as dramatic or as restrained as you like. You also have the option of curling your hair or leaving it straight. All you need is a hair clip, two hair bands, some hair grips and a comb.

1. Take a 5cm (2in) section from directly behind one ear and clip the rest of your hair out of the way for now.

2. Create a simple plait with the small section, then secure it with a hair band. If you want to keep the plait lying flat against your head, overdirecting it upwards while you work will help. Create a matching plait on the other side.

3. Take a vertical section of hair, a little way back from your hairline, and backcomb aggressively at the roots.

4. Continue backcombing vertical sections of hair in this way until you've achieved the desired volume.

5. Now drape each plait across your head, a few centimetres away from your hairline, and secure them behind the ears with hair grips.

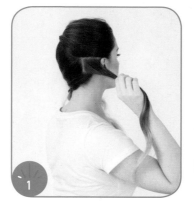

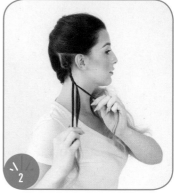

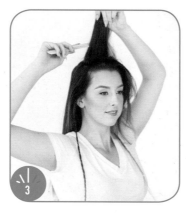

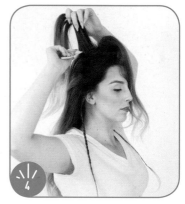

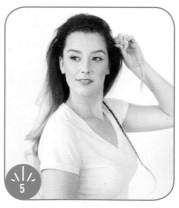

tip

If your hair is resistant to back-combing, create a better hold by adding some dry shampoo to the roots before you begin.

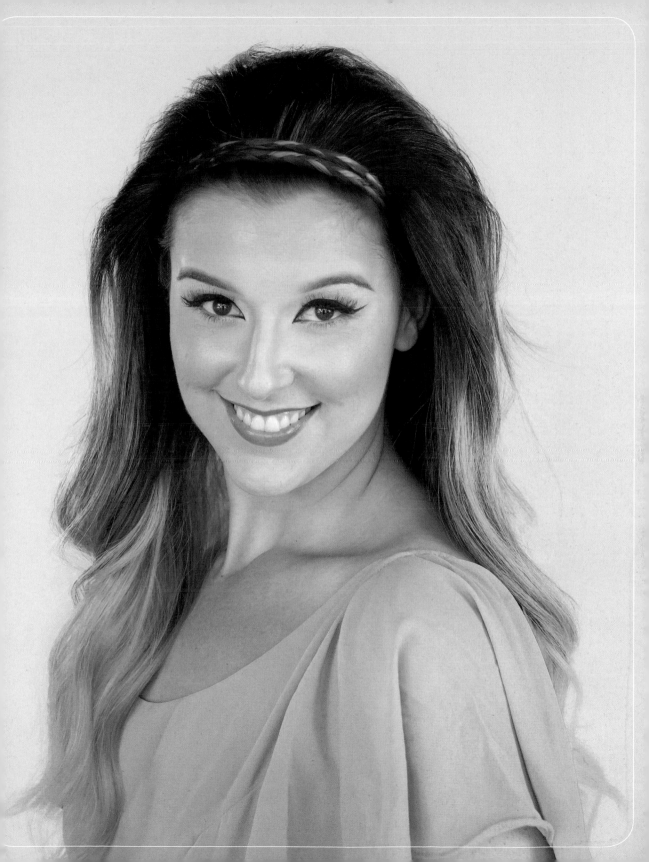

BACKCOMB AND TIE

As long as you have hair long enough to tie into a knot, then you can accomplish this awesome look! This is one of the easiest styles you can choose, and it's perfect for when you fancy an unfussy, casual look. You simply backcomb your hair at the roots with a comb, add a bit of hairspray or texturizing spray, then tie two strands of hair together behind your head.

1. Working from the high crown to the low crown, take small sections of hair and backcomb the roots of each one in turn.

2. When the backcombing is complete, lightly comb over the top of it to create a clean-textured layer of hair on the surface.

3. Now grab a 2.5–5cm (1–2in) section from above your ear on both sides of your head.

4. Bring these two sections of hair to the back of your head, and tie them together in the low-nape area. Tie a second knot underneath the first knot.

5. To give a little bit of extra security, attach a hair band underneath both knots to hold them in place.

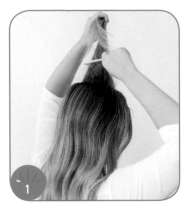

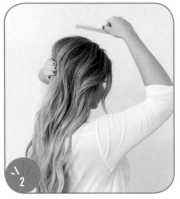

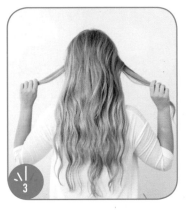

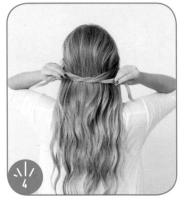

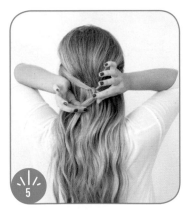

tip

If you have silky hair, add a pomade to the side sections prior to tying. This will help the style last all day!

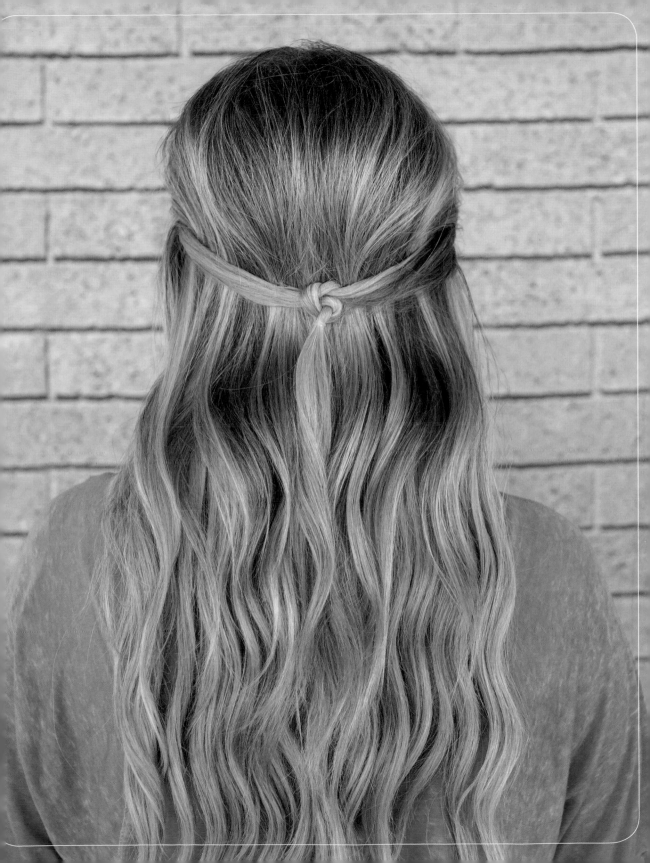

SIDESWEPT PINBACK

The sideswept pinback is a great style on everyone and on all hair lengths, and with only a few simple steps, you'll be on your way out the door in less than five minutes. Like many of the other styles in this book, this is an incredibly versatile look, too – keep it casual for work, or glamorous for a night out! All you need to have to hand is a comb, curling tongs, a hair clip and a hair grip or two.

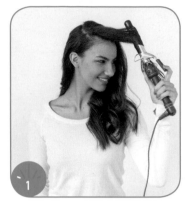

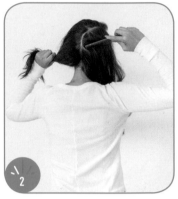

1. Prep your hair before styling by working through any tangles you may have and adding a light curl with your curling tongs. You don't need to spend much time on this – just a few strands is fine.

2. Part your hair to the desired side, working from your hairline down to the nape of your neck.

3. Clip the larger section out of the way for now.

4. Take the smaller section of hair and twist it towards the far side of your neck. Secure this hair in place using a hair grip.

5. Now release the clipped-away section of hair. Re-curl any strands that may have loosened too much in the meantime, and then finish off the whole look with hairspray.

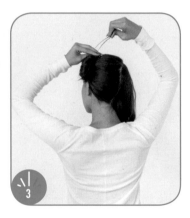

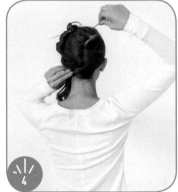

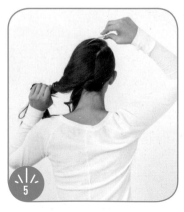

tip

You can change this whole look just by the way you prep your hair prior to styling. For a casual look, go with straight hair, or add glamour with tight curls.

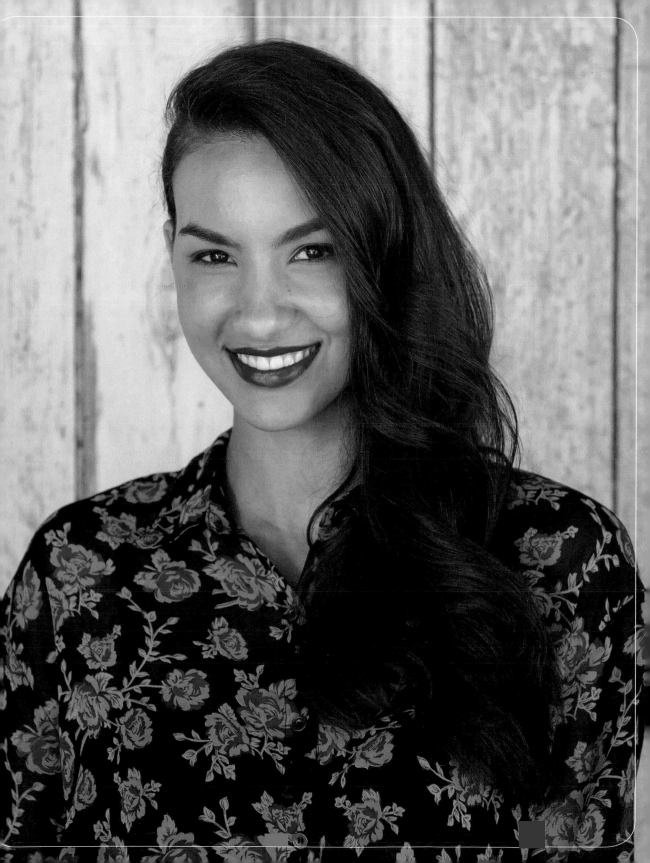

TWIST AND PUSH-UP STYLE

Not only can this classic hairstyle be created in minutes, it can also be worn anywhere and everywhere. You can backcomb your roots and curl your hair before you begin styling for a more formal look, or you can begin with natural hair if you want to keep it looking modest and minimal for everyday wear. You will need just a comb and a few hair grips to hold everything in place.

1. Part your hair if desired and then divide your hair in half horizontally, from ear to ear.

2. Pull your hair back towards the low-crown area, then begin rotating the hair with your hand, creating a slight French twist.

3. Now push the twisted hair upwards so that you create more volume in the crown.

4. Secure the twist in place with a few hair grips. On the right side of the twist, grab the hair with the lip of a hair grip, then rotate and push the grip into the twist, directing it upwards.

5. Add just a bit more volume and texture to finish off by gently holding on to the base of your twist while you pull carefully at the hair around the top of your head.

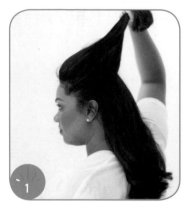

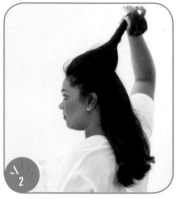

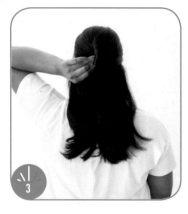

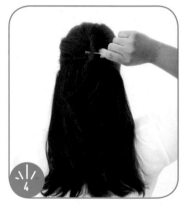

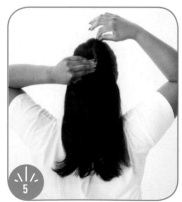

tip

If you have thin hair, or you just don't want to backcomb, try blow-drying with a volumising mousse before starting.

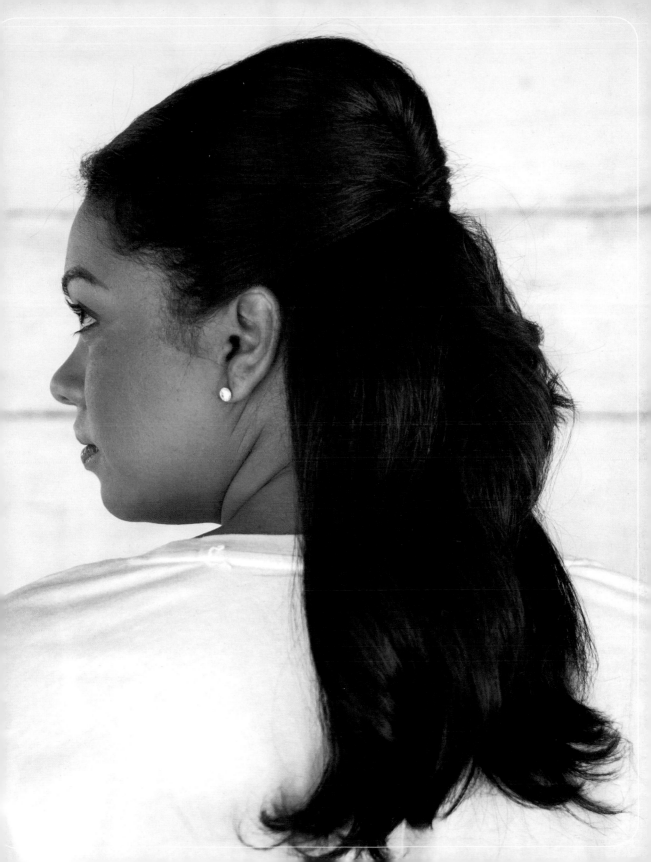

DOUBLE TWISTS INTO SIMPLE PLAIT

This five-minute style is great for summer, and you can make it as simple or as complicated as you want. For instance, instead of twisting your hair, you could simply plait it. This hairstyle is ideal for those of you with minimal layering in your hair, but if you do have a lot of layers, simply curl before starting. You'll need a hair band, a hair clip and a comb to hand before you begin.

1. On each side of your head, separate out a large triangular section (roughly 5–8cm/ 2–3in wide).

2. Twist the hair in each triangular section away from your face and down at an angle, towards the lower back of your head.

3. Connect both twists at the back and clip them together for later. Now divide all of your hair into three equal sections. Keeping the twists clipped together, create a three-strand plait, incorporating the hair emerging from the twists.

4. Plait your hair until you reach the ends, then secure them with a hair band.

5. Finish off by removing the clip from the twists, then 'pancake' the plait to create more fullness.

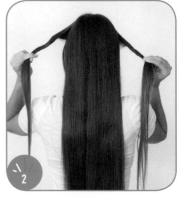

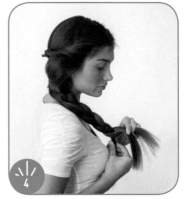

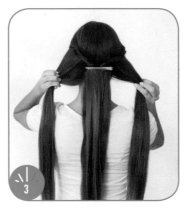

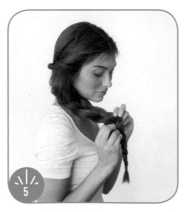

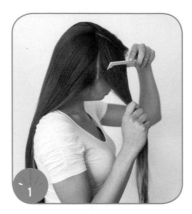

tip

For a more textured and bohemian look, create this style on naturally curly or previously curled hair.

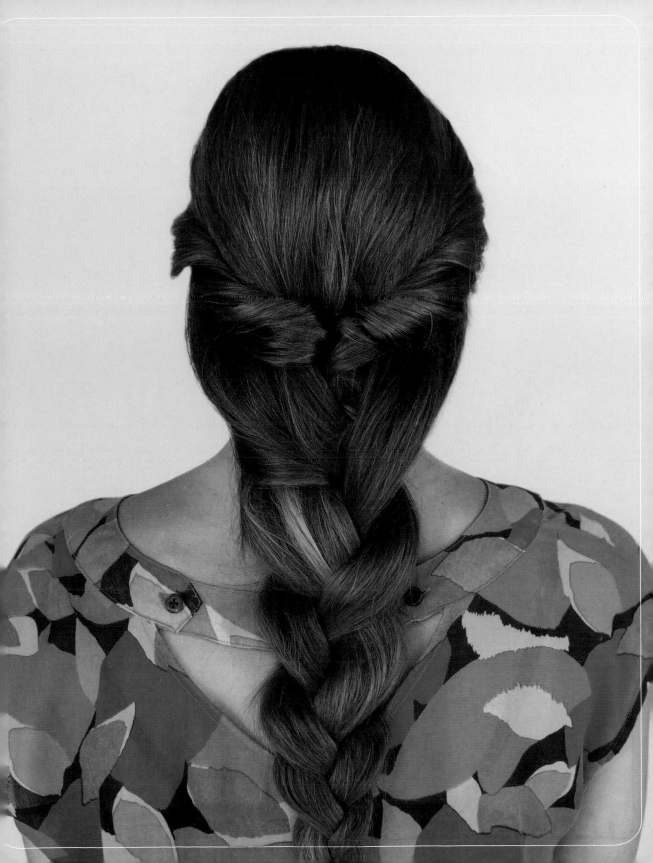

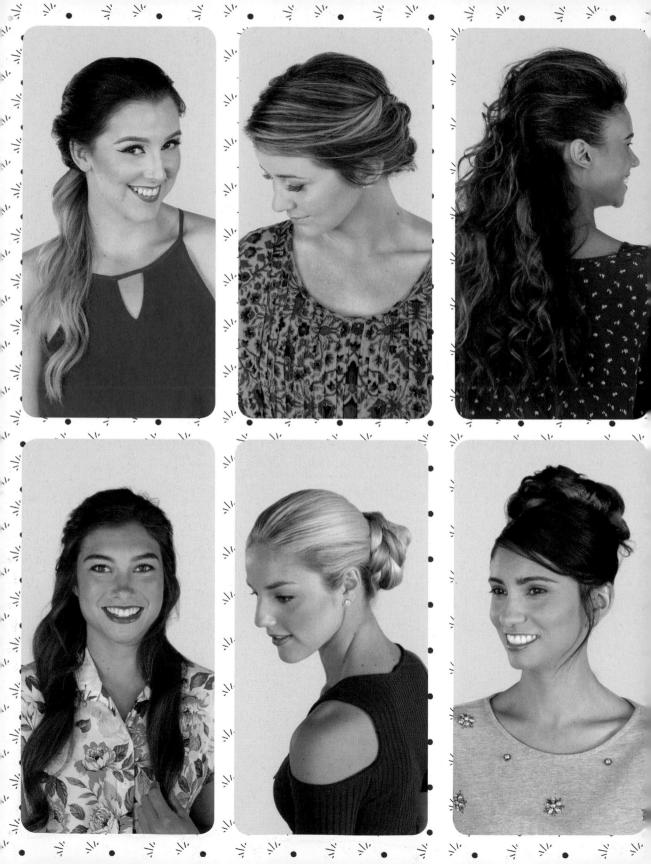

6

Resources

TOOLS

Blow-dryer
A styling tool that, in addition to drying hair, is great for adding volume or for smoothing and straightening out hair.

Curling tongs
A styling tool that uses heat to create a consistent curl on a portion of hair.

Dry shampoo
A hairstyling product that helps give greasy or second-day hair a freshly-washed look. It is also a good product for adding texture to hair before styling.

Straighteners
A styling tool that uses heat between two metal plates in order to take hair from curly to straight.

Hair band
A rubber band that gathers and secures hair in the form of a ponytail. It is also used to secure the ends of the hair – for example, with plaits.

Hair clip
This is a large clip used to hold sections of hair out of the way while you work on another section.

Hair extension
Synthetic or real human hair woven together on a hair weft that you can attach to your own natural hair to add length or volume. There are several different types of extensions for temporary use that can be attached using glue or tape, protein bonded or clipped in.

Hair grip
These are used to hold sections of hair in place. (For larger sections of hair, such as buns, you can also use longer hair pins, rather than hair grips.)

Paddle brush
A flat brush that can be used to detangle, straighten and flatten hair. It can also be used to tame flyaways.

Pomade
A water-based substance that is used to style hair and set styles. It does not dry out the hair and leaves it looking shiny and slick.

Serum
A thicker shine product that helps with flyaways.

Shine spray
A product that adds shine to frizzy hair.

Texturising spray
A product that adds texture to the hair.

Volumising mousse
Also referred to as styling foam, this product is used to give the hair more shine and volume. It is often used while blow-drying the hair.

Low bun with plaited headband variation, pages 80-81

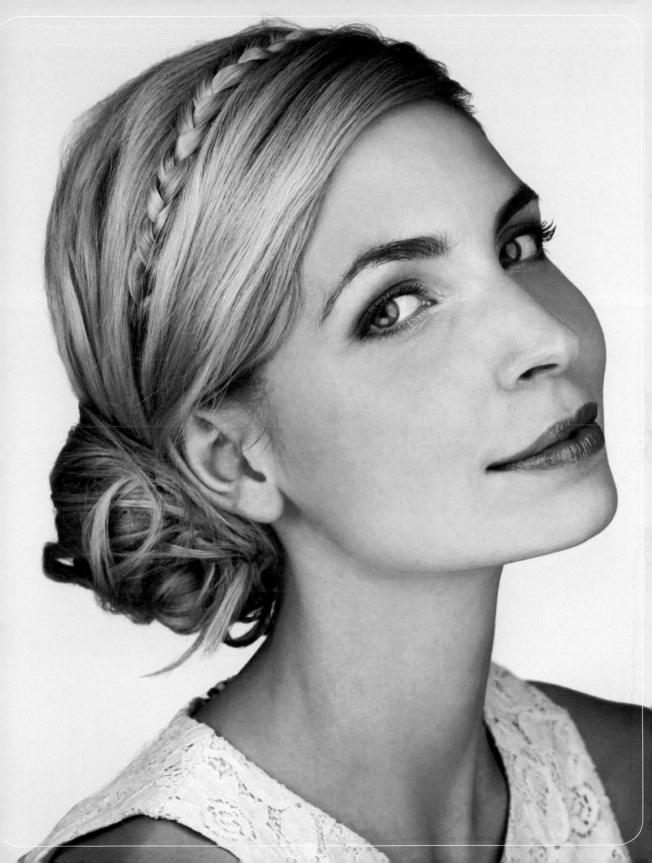

GLOSSARY

Backcombing
A technique that uses a comb to reverse-brush the hair (in the direction of the roots) in order to create long-lasting volume. (Also known as 'teasing'.)

Crown
The upper back portion of your head.

Dutch plait
A three-strand technique that crosses sections under one another, while also drawing hair in from either side of the plait in turn. Similar to a French plait, but in this case the resulting plait sits on top of the hair.

Fishtail plait
A two-strand technique that criss-crosses small strands of hair alternately, overlapping two larger sections, to create a thick plait with a densely woven appearance.

French plait
A three-strand technique that crosses sections of hair over one another, while also incorporating hair from

either side of the plait. Unlike the Dutch plait, the French plait has an inverted appearance, due to the over-and-under movement of the strands.

High crown
The highest point of the crown on the back of the head.

Hairline
The hair that grows along the perimeter of your head, including around your face and along your neckline.

Hair section
A portion of hair that is clipped back while you work on other sections.

Low crown
Several centimetres above the nape of the neck.

Nape
The area where your hairline meets your neck.

Pancake
This is the act of pulling and stretching out the strands of a plait so as to create additional volume.

Plait
Also referred to as a braid, a technique that involves weaving sections of hair into each other. There are several ways you can plait your hair, including three-strand plaits, Dutch plaits, French plaits and fishtail plaits.

Round-brushing
Round brushes are good for creating curls. They also add grip while blow-drying so you are able to give the hair a sleeker finish.

Towel-drying
A method of drying the hair with a towel. When towel-drying, the hair should be squeezed through the towel, rather than rubbed, to avoid causing split ends.

Side fishtail bun, pages 36-37

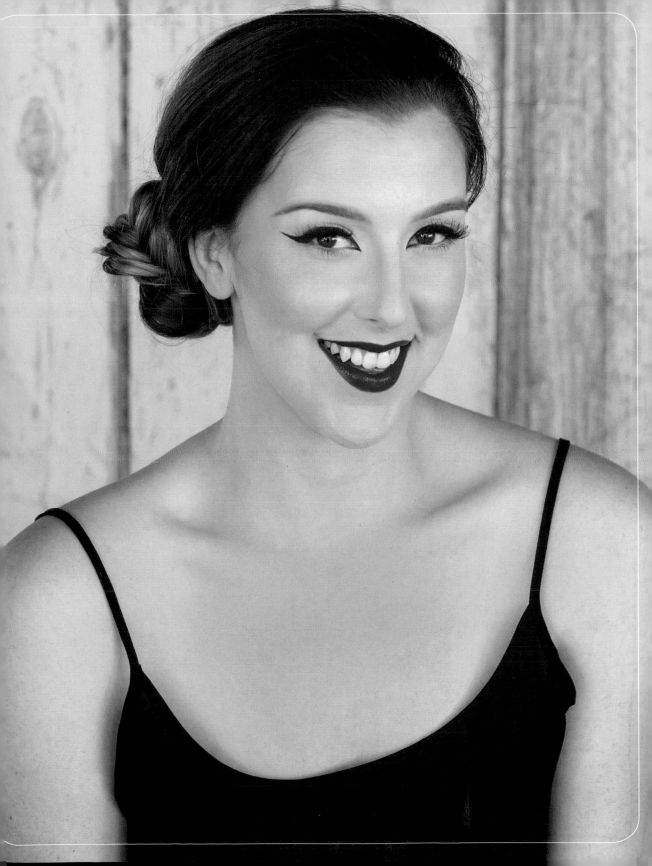

CONTRIBUTOR CREDITS

Contributing editor and make-up
Cheyenne Folkert

All photography
Sara Bishop

Getty Images
(pages 121, 125)

Author's assistant
Emily Armijo

Models
Shelby Barnes
(pages 10–11, 38–39, 54–55, 70–71, 102–103)

Brianna Byars
(pages 88–89, 114–115)

Shireen Dooling
(pages 12–13, 72–73, 76–77, 86–87)

Cheyenne Folkert
(pages 16–17, 20–21, 36–37, 62–63, 108–109, 123)

Angela Gutierrez
(pages 6, 22–23, 40–41, 50–51, 64–65, 116–117)

Jasmine Jacobson
(pages 26–27, 60–61, 74–75, 104–105)

Mallory Jarvis
(pages 42–43, 52–53, 94–95)

Bryce May
(pages 28–29, 68–69, 90–91, 106–107)

Dominique Muscianese
(pages 14–15, 30–31, 48–49, 112–113)

Ashley Petty
(pages 80–81, 96–97, 110–111)

Alexia Poisot
(pages 18–19, 46–47, 82–83)

Jacque Stuard
(pages 24–25, 34–35, 44–45, 66–67)

Lacy Urban
(pages 58–59, 78–79, 92–93, 98–99)

WEBSITES

Jenny Strebe
theconfessionsofahairstylist.com

Other blogs
abeautifulmess.com

curlynikki.com

freckled-fox.com

hairandmakeupbysteph.com

hairromance.com

maneaddicts.com

missysue.com

thesmallthingsblog.com

twistmepretty.com

Training
Aveda Institutes
aveda.edu

Toni and Guy
Hairdressing Academytoniguy.edu

Vidal Sassoon Academy
sassoon-academy.com

Paul Mitchell
paulmitchell.edu

Regency Beauty Institute
regency.edu

Sharon Blain
sharonblain.com

Simple three-strand plait

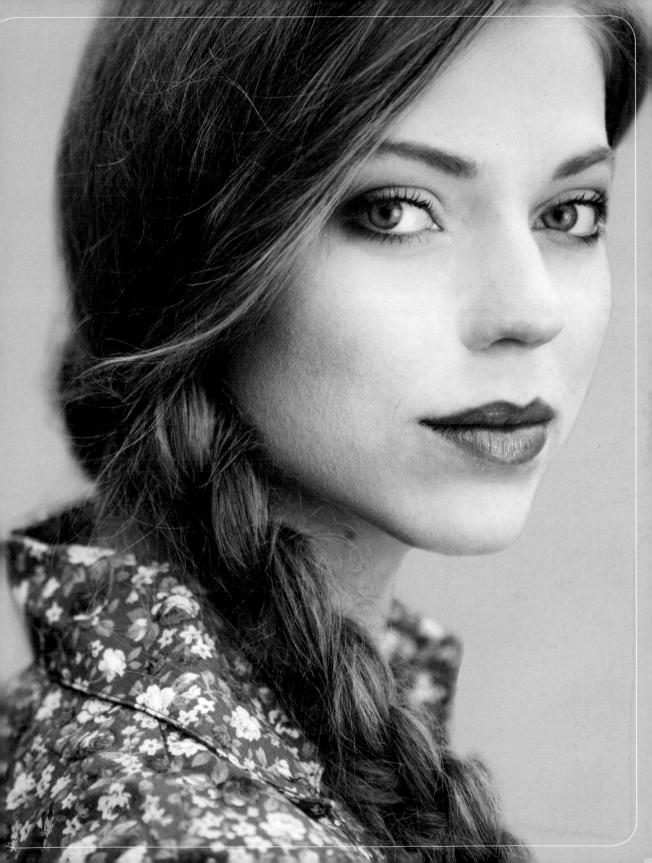

INDEX

ACKNOWLEDGEMENTS

This book has been an absolute dream to work on, thanks to my incredible support team, who have so kindly donated their talents and time to making it all happen.

The first of many thanks has to go to my supportive husband, Casey, whose constant love, patience and encouragement has given me the strength to pursue my passion. You are my rock.

To my kids – your unconditional love means everything to me and helps me face the many challenges along the way. Thanks for always being my number-one fans.

A massive thank you to my photographer, Sara Bishop. You are an absolute star and super-talented woman. I was so grateful to have you in my corner, as always.

To my awesome rockstar editor, Angela Koo, who was an absolute joy to work with, and whose patience was outstanding. We couldn't have kept to the deadlines without you!

And lastly, a huge thank you to my writing assistant, Cheyenne Folkert, because without her patience during all of our photoshoots, and her putting my technical steps into beautiful words, this book just wouldn't be the same.